AIDS, God, and Faith

Continuing the Dialogue on Constructing Gay Theology

Ronald E. Long, Ph.D.
J. Michael Clark, Ph.D.

Las Colinas
Monument Press
1992

Published by
Monument Press
Las Colinas, Texas

This is Supplemental Volume 2 in the Gay Men's Issues in Religious Studies, Proceedings of the Gay Men's Issues in Religion Consultation of the American Academy of Religion.

Copyright 1992, Monument Press

Library of Congress Cataloging-in-Publication Data

Long, Ronald E (Ronald Edwin), 1946-
    AIDS, God, and faith : continuing the dialogue on constructing gay theology / Ronald E. Long, J. Michael Clark.
        p. cm.
    Supplement to: Constructing gay theology.
    "Gay men's issues in religious studies, volume 2, supplement."
    Includes bibliographical references and index.
    ISBN 0-930383-25-7 : $7.00
    1. Homosexuality--Religious aspects--Christianity. 2. AIDS (Disease)--Religious aspects--Christianity. 3. Gay men--Religious life. 4. Liberation theology. 5. Theodicy. I. Clark, J. Michael (John Michael), 1953-   . II. Gay men's issues in religious studies. V. 2 (Supplement) III. Title. IV. Title: Constructing gay theology.
BR115.H6C68 1991 Suppl.
261.8'35766--dc20
                                                            92-18829
                                                                CIP

Table of Contents

The authors of the present volume wish to thank the
Gay Men's Issues in Religion Group, American Academy of Religion,
for providing the forum in which this dialogue was begun
and for providing the empowerment by which it continues.

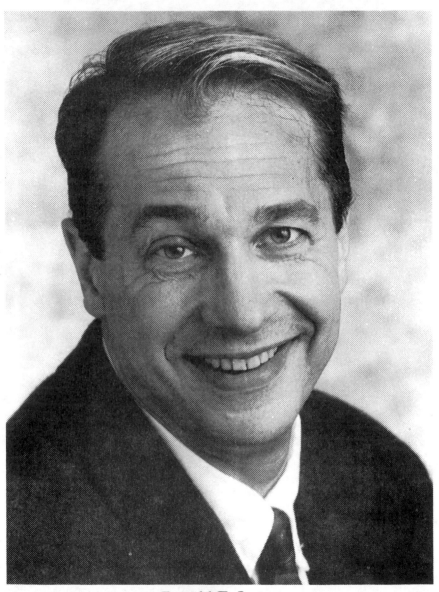

Ronald E. Long

I. God Through Gay Men's Eyes:
Gay Theology in the Age of AIDS
Ronald E. Long, PH.D.

The following reflections are offered *in memoriam* for **James R. Brewer** (1951-1986), my lover of nine years.

When the works of the prophets of Ancient Israel were included in the biblical canon, the recognition that religion could become dysfunctional became part of the Western religious heritage. For prophets like Amos, neither piety nor observance could guarantee a right relation with God if social justice were lacking. The charge of Amos is but an early variant on a recurrent theme: when religion supplants or diffuses the task of moral maturation, it fails to function religiously. Ideally, religion is that cultural enterprise through which human beings envision and seek to nurture their essential humanization. When religion asks us to deny, suppress, or condemn what can only be renounced at the risk of self-betrayal, it has become dysfunctional. As such, it will be--and ought to be--abandoned, superseded, or transformed.

At this juncture in time, these are the options with which the gay community is faced. To be gay is to accept a homosexual--or more precisely, a homophilic--orientation as essential to who one is *and* to refuse to consent to shame about it. To the extent traditional religion devalues the sense of self and world which a gay person can compromise only at the risk of self-betrayal, it has ceased to perform religiously. Fidelity to gay experience in our day--in the age of AIDS--may thus require us to abandon or radically reenvision our religious heritage.

Traditional Western religion continues to fail the gay community in at least two important respects. Gay men and lesbians cannot help but be relegated to marginal status in mainline communities of faith. The continued resistance to the ordination of openly gay individuals on the part of most mainline traditions, both Jewish and Christian, is testimony to the continued hold of the idea that God and homosexual being and behavior are mutually antagonistic realities. Secondly, belief in the personal, loving God of tradition is strained by the radical evil which is AIDS. While AIDS is not explicitly a "gay" disease, gay men have been especially hit hard by it. The presence of AIDS among us, like all catastrophic events, raises in a particularly acute form the problem of evil: whether it is logical or, more importantly, credible that evil (much less, so much evil) should exist in a world created and providentially ordered by a God who is omniscient, omnipotent, and absolutely good.

The two issues are conjoined in an insidious way when it is claimed, as has been done popularly, that AIDS is a God-sent punishment for homosexuality. Apparently for some, God must so hate homosexuals and their sexual behavior that he is provoked to visit them with a dire disease, while he is content to let rapists and child molesters and murderers remain hale and healthy. Such a god surely has a skewed sense of proportion. We have been taught to think of God as good, indeed as absolutely good. Yet, if we insist on seeing AIDS as punishment from God, we risk attributing actions to God that, when attributed to a man, would constitute human immorality. And must not a god be at least as good as a man to merit worship? It was on behalf of a more viable view of God that the late David Summers would claim that, if God is to be said to have sent

AIDS--and that is bad theology at best--then AIDS must be seen, not as punishment, but as an occasion to love.[1]

Summer's insight leaves us with a further question: if it is bad theology to think of God as the "sender" of AIDS, then what would good theology look like? In particular, how might gay experience lead one to speak of God? In short, what would a viable gay theology look like? Much energy has been lavished upon exorcising the divide between the God of tradition and homosexuality in an attempt to defuse the homophobia of biblical and doctrinal sources. It is on the problem of evil, however, that gay belief must falter in the age of AIDS: no gay who is in touch with the radical evil which is AIDS should give his worshipful devotion to a God who is in any way responsible for that disease which lays waste his friends and lovers. Only a thorough reconstruction of the idea of God can finally commend itself for morally sensitive gay belief.

(i)

Inadequate reconstruction of the idea of God haunts the otherwise admirable contributions of John McNeill[2] and John Fortunato.[3] McNeill's *Taking a Chance on God* is, in many respects, a wise, important, and heroic book. The publication of his views--challenging, as they do, official Catholic teaching--has already resulted in his expulsion from the Society of Jesus. The so-called Halloween Letter issued by the Vatican in 1988 describes homosexuality as an "objective disorder" "tending" towards immorality;[4] in short, the homosexual is disordered even if he is totally celibate. Against this, *Taking a Chance on God* attempts to outline a spirituality for gays rooted in the conviction already sounded in the earlier *The Church and the Homosexual*, namely, that a gay orientation is so much a part of one's being--not just one's doing--that to grasp one's homosexuality as an "objective disorder" is to find oneself a mistake, damaged goods, a freak--a view psychologically as well as spiritually damning. Rather, McNeill bids the gay individual to "take a chance on God," to dare to think that God knows what he is doing in creating gay persons, to assume that one's homosexuality has a point within the divine scheme of things. And the book itself tries to spell out what living out that risk would entail. Therein lies the book's wisdom.

However, McNeill is characteristically comfortable in talking of a God who intends and has plans--and in understanding events and realities in terms of their point within the divine purpose. And it is the credibility of such talk that the reality of AIDS strains. An appendix to the third edition of *The Church and the Homosexual* is McNeill's most extended treatment of the issue of AIDS.[5] There he very firmly states that God does not *intend* that any particular person be afflicted with AIDS. (Whether God might, in willing or allowing AIDS in general, will AIDS for an individual *unintentionally* remains an undiscussed point.) Having said that, he moves directly to a discussion of why AIDS is not a punishment sent from God. Apparently, if God intended for any particular person to have AIDS, it could not be other than as a punishment. But it is against the idea that AIDS might be a punishment from God that McNeill directs his animus. To believe that God punishes in this way is, for McNeill, ultimately un-Christian: it is to acknowledge a fearful, not a loving, god, a god other than the "Father" of Jesus of Nazareth. McNeill points out that the *Gospel of John* (9:2-3) has it that, when asked whether a given man's physical afflictions were the result of his own or his parents' sin, Jesus answers "Neither":

> The mistake made by Jesus' friends here was in assuming a direct cause and effect connection between one's moral choices and one's circumstances. Jesus points out that reality is not

that simple: he speaks of a God who lets the sun shine on the good and the bad alike and who gives rain to those who do good as well as those who do evil.[6]

Yet AIDS is with us. And, if AIDS is not a punishment from God, it presumably has a place in God's plan. It could be argued, of course, that evils such as AIDS might not be preventable, even by God.[7] But such a claim would represent a challenge to the omnipotence of God and thereby to the classical theism McNeill seems otherwise to assume. Indeed, McNeill's entire agenda involves the accommodation of a gay identity within a traditional Catholic mythos. If God could prevent AIDS, but chooses not to do so, then AIDS must be by God's consent and must ultimately serve God's goal or purpose. That is, God must will AIDS in general either because AIDS can rise to good or because it might be necessary for the emergence of some good. At this point, McNeill retreats to the hope that AIDS will prove to have served some good. When he dares to speculate on what good could possibly be the excuse for AIDS, he relies upon the insights of John Fortunato.

In Fortunato's work *AIDS, the Spiritual Dilemma*,[8] the conflict between the reality of AIDS and belief in God is brought into high relief and, despite Fortunato's own attempts at reconciliation, traditional belief reveals its inadequacy. Fortunato argues, and rightly I think, that the impact of AIDS upon the gay community is particularly troubling because of the sense of self that a gay identity inevitably bears. A gay identity is one that is constellated around the direction of a person's sexual desiring. Since gay desire is homophilic, procreation is not its "excuse" for being. What passes for homophobia should, Fortunato argues, be more fully understood as "erotophobia," fear of sexual desire in particular, and of desire itself in general-- for the homosexual represents an identity in which desire for pleasure is acknowledged and confessed, not as accidental, but as essential to human self-hood. This is troubling in a culture born of Christianity's appropriation of an alien Greek dualism in which spirit is pitted against nature, mind over matter, and reason over against passion. Where sanctity is recognized as self-control, desire must be distrusted and renounced along with the world and the devil. At best, one can allow oneself to be carried away with the "desires of the flesh" only for legitimate reason, to have a baby for example. In America, where lust seems to many not one of the deadly sins, but sin itself, it is no wonder that the homosexual draws down upon himself the charge of decadence and immorality.

Those who take their sexual orientation as a central element of their identity cannot help but take their bodies as an essential element of their personhood as well. The philosopher Marcel repeatedly argued, while a person may be more than his or her body, it is more appropriate to say that one "is" rather than "has" a body. To know the self as sexed is to know the self as embodied, as animated body rather than soul imprisoned in flesh. Fortunato sees embodiment, moreover, not only as a general truth of the human condition, but a Christian truth as well: the Church, in opting to express itself in the language of Greek dualism, opted for an un-Biblical, and hence "heretical," view of the body. Thus, the homosexual is daring to witness to a Christian truth in a culture that holds instead to a Greek heresy. However that may be, it is precisely because of the gay testimony to human embodiment that AIDS is so poignant and distressing. If gays dare to show the human as essentially body, then AIDS proves the body--and the self--to be mortal. The homosexual comes to represent not only desire, then, but also death. The fear of death fuels fear of the gay, turning straight against gay and gay against gay, and tempts the gay man himself to internalize the culture's homophobia and renounce his gayness. A gay identity and the gay witness to humanity's essential embodiment can be sustained, argues Fortunato, only as we some-how become reconciled to our own mortality; and this, in turn, can only be accomplished as we are able to give up our dead and die ourselves *in hope*. Ultimately, for Fortu-nato, AIDS represents a challenge for the gay community to win through to something he calls "resurrection hope", a hope that the death of anyone (metaphorical or real) not be the final reality about them--that there is a future even for the dead. Fortunato does not entertain the thought that such hope may be the substance of faith; rather, he chooses to think that hope is the *result* of belief in an omniscient, om-nipotent, omni-benevolent God. It strains credibility, how-ever, to suppose that a god who would send AIDS could be trusted to provide a future even for the dead.

Fortunato refuses to compromise on God's omnipo-tence (God could prevent AIDS), God's omniscience (God knows the full impact of his actions), or God's goodness (God does not have a mean streak)--as others have done. And he readily admits to bafflement when he tries to rec-oncile the idea of an all-good creator god with the stark re-ality of the physical disintegration and disfigurement, the social and psychological ugliness, which is AIDS. In the absence of any rational justification for AIDS, Fortunato retreats from intellectualist engagement with the problem of evil and suggests treating the idea of God and the reality of AIDS as two elements in a koan.[9] In Zen practice, a koan, like the question "What is the sound of one hand clapping?," is supposed to exacerbate the natural human in-clination to substitute thought for direct responsiveness and cause the mind to "burn out" so that only an unfettered re-sponsiveness remains. Just so, argues Fortunato, the thought of God and a world of AIDS, resistant to a fully acceptable intellectual harmonization, really causes the be-liever to give up on thinking and respond with an unfet-tered charity. The suggestion is ingenious. However, the suggestion finally undermines the importance of belief in

God. If the point of the "koan of evil" is to bring forth charity, belief--like the Zen koan itself--is ultimately to be left behind, transcended, for the koan is but a vehicle. And, since no one would want to say belief is a *necessary* vehicle for the emergence of "charity," belief reveals its expendability.

Further analysis reveals the moral problem with belief. Finally confessing that he has no rational solution to the problem of "why AIDS?," Fortunato nevertheless attempts a "non-rational" answer: the meaning of AIDS, that which gives some excuse for its existence, lies precisely in its being an instrument for the awakening of our awareness and acceptance of our own mortality--AIDS exists as a stimulus to an authentic faith.[10] Such a position is too reminiscent of the position of the priest in Camus' novel *The Plague*[11] not to invite comparison. The novel itself is an account of a bubonic-like plague that strikes the residents of a fictional Oran that results in quarantine and massive death before it surprisingly disappears. Fr. Paneloux, the novel's spokesman for what Camus ultimately thought of as the religious position, gives two sermons in the course of the novel. In the first, Paneloux struggles with the question of what point the plague must have, concluding that the plague must be a stimulus for conversion. Camus' novel operates on several levels at once. On one level, the story of the plague is a story about the plague of Fascism which enveloped pre-World War II Europe and the plague of Stalinist dictatorship. More extensively, it serves to indict any system which, in Camus' terms, "justifies" murder. In context, then, the sermon of Paneloux serves to put God in the position of a Fascist leader who violates the flesh so that faith may abound. Such a divine ruler is, in Camus' novel, but an almighty dictatorial murderer.

Perhaps we have reached a point when talk about God has outlived its usefulness and ought simply to be abandoned--especially in an era when the Cardinal O'Con-

nors and Jerry Falwells of this world are held up as religious authorities. Perhaps the gay community ought to let
God, religion, and theology die a quiet death and move on
to the business of caring for its own and advancing its own
agenda. Perhaps, however, both theology and talk about
God are not so easily left aside. Perhaps they serve a function that it is unwise to neglect. McNeill writes that gay
atheism, the rejection of religion and the idea of God, may
be a psychological necessity for many to come to maturity:

> For most of my clients the idea of God became so identified
> with homophobic self-hatred that the only way they could deal
> with God was to take a vacation from religion while they dealt
> with the process of coming out and accepting themselves.
> Only after they had a secure, positive self-image were they
> able to make a critical return to the question of religious be-
> lief.[12]

Just as McNeill opens the possibility of a religion which is
no longer childish religion, perhaps we must entertain the
possibility that there are mature ways of speaking to the divine. At least one is tempted to explore the question of
whether being gay in the age of AIDS involves a faith and,
if so, whether one could speak of God in its light.

(ii)

Whatever God may be in Godself, we relate to God
as we have been taught to think of "him."[13] We perceive
deity according to the ideas about God that are regnant in
our culture. The fact is, the idea of God is the residuum of
a long historical development--it is an idea which has been
forged in history and thus has the status of a cultural construct. But what has been constructed is subject to reconstruction, what has once been envisioned can be re-envi-
sioned.

In point of fact, the ongoing revision of the idea of God is part of what constitutes our religious heritage. While it may have been "natural" for an early Hebrew society to think of its God as caring for it by championing its cause in war against other peoples and their gods, the prophets had to rethink what kind of care Israel's God really exercised if he was content to use the Assyrians to destroy the very nation he championed. So, too, the early Christians had to rethink what the "fatherhood" of God must have meant if this "Father" could let his "Son" be executed as a criminal. Today, the Jewish community is attempting to rethink the idea of God in a post-Holocaust world. So, too, as gay men, we are summoned to take up the mantle of tradition and rethink the idea of God in the light of our experience--post-Stonewall, post-HIV.

But how do we proceed? No one takes it as anything other than poetic license to speak of God as walking around on the earth as portions of *Genesis* do. Whatever God might be, God is not a being within experience like another person. There is no figure "God" in our experience to whom we can turn to verify our ideas about "him" like we can turn to George to check out our ideas about George.

However, the word "God" principally refers to that reality which anchors our sense of what is truly important. While we do, from time to time, change our lifestyle according to how we come to see the world, coming to see the world religiously--coming to believe in God--is above all a matter of coming to accept the fit of the value commitments that the idea of God supports. Two methodological points follow. The first is negative: God cannot be conceived in any way that would conflict with our deepest value commitments. For example, from the perspective of gay theology, to speak of God in any way that would imply that God either "sends" or even merely "tolerates" AIDS is morally anathema. Positively, God for us will be the god revealed as we unpack the wider affirmations about the world implicit in the establishment of a gay identity. While there might be a number of "worlds" which would prove hospitable to a gay identity, gay theology proper is the specification of the world implied in the affirmation of the self as gay. And analysis of the gay commitment reveals a reality that can legitimately be called "God," although that god is not the god of theism.

But why bother doing theology at all? Why bother envisioning the world religiously? The enterprise of gay theology is ultimately justified as an act of profound self-understanding and self clarification. It gains further justification from the practical edge that one gains by knowing what it is we may in fact be about. Avoidance of self-understanding is irresponsible--and, although self-understanding of ourselves as gay in the age of AIDS may reveal that we are alienated from the god of traditional theism, we may not be cut off from the divine. If I am right, the gay community can have both theology and God.

(iii)

The decisive act for all gay persons is the act of "coming out." Coming out is not really a single action, but a complex series of acts that can be arrayed on a continuum running from the recognition of one's homoerotic desires as a permanent and important aspect of oneself to the decision to identify oneself as gay publicly to family, friends, colleagues, etc. The recognition of homoeroticism as essential to oneself, that one cannot deny it without ceasing to be vitally the self that one is, is the decisive moment, and takes not a little courage in a culture that sees such desiring itself, whether it issues in action or not, as abnormal. Coming out is thus a mode of self-affirmation in the face of whatever would frustrate essential self-definition and self-expression. In this light, gay theology might be tempted to develop in an essentially Tillichian direction: coming out, as an act of courageous self-affirmation and thus an epiphany of the courage-to-be, would be a matter of getting caught up in the eternal rhythm by which being overcomes non-being, that is, to be grounded in the divine life itself.

However, this is an age in which HIV infection has come among us. To admit even to oneself that one is gay in the age of AIDS is not merely to identify oneself as having a variant sexual orientation, but it is to align oneself (even if only by identification and through no further action) with a community that is especially hard hit by, and especially active in the fight against, HIV infection. It is a community that knows itself to be locked in a battle. One need only note the preference for martial imagery in its literature.[14]   Plague is among us and, in the age of AIDS, coming out as a gay person is to find oneself defined as a part of a community which is in the forefront in that resistance movement which is the fight against AIDS. And in battle, victory, not the fight, is the point.

My language is intentionally evocative of the imagery of Camus' *The Rebel*[15] and *The Plague.* The works taken together advocate a life of clarity, where clarity involves both the full realization of the evilness of victimization and oppression and the awareness of the myriad ways in which such victimization occurs--whether the source be natural, social, or divine, whether we are in complicity or not. The life of clarity is thus grounded in an anger with oppressive victimization and issues in battle, as well as in a refusal of complicity, with victimization, evil, and death.

And it is the anger of the gay community that cannot be missed. Anger at the physical suffering of the sick. Anger over their disablement and disfigurement. Anger over their psychological turmoil--and that of the merely infected, as well as the "worried well." Anger that AIDS has put many of our lives on hold as we go about the day-to-day work of caring for our sick. Anger over a state that was, and is, slow to come to our aid as our lovers and friends are dying. Anger that saving medicines are with-held in the name of pure investigative rigor. Anger that drug companies can truly capitalize on our misfortune. The list goes on. And our anger finally bellows out the cry that AIDS has no excuse for being. It is in anguished indigna-tion that we cry out that AIDS should never have been or ever should exist.

Ruben Alves, the Brazilian theologian, has argued that the gut conviction that any particular instance of suf-fering ought under no circumstance to be or to have been is really to appeal to God, for God is to be defined as that re-ality which guarantees that our feelings of revulsion at any given evil are more than my, or even our, parochial feel-ings.[16] Here he follows a long tradition of thinking that has argued that man's ability to judge this or that facet of experience as good or bad is to be in contact with the di-vine. St. Augustine had argued, for example, that it is only our taste for perfection that enables us to judge the relative perfections within experience, and that our taste for perfec-tion is none other than our "taste" for God. Unfortunately, these various interpretations severally tend to put us into contact with the personal, agentic God of tradition, belief in which is so problematic for a community suffering from AIDS.

One might want to see each of these arguments as philosophical variations on the doctrine that man was cre-ated in the image of God where man is in God's image in virtue of his moral constitution. To indulge in anthropo-morphic imagery for a moment, man's passionate protest over injustice and compassion for its victims is an echo of the divine pathos. But the real question is who is created in the image of whom? Does God create man in his image, or does man image God after himself? The genius of our in-herited traditions lies in the discovery of the human-heartedness of the divine, generally concluding that hu-mans should therefore defer to the divine, understood as

"God," in obedience in matters moral and in trust in matters existential, for God knows more than we do and really has our best interests at heart. But, perhaps, the time has come to recognize, not the human-like character of the divine, but the godliness of the human heart. The tradition has it that God is love, but the tradition has been reluctant to affirm the reverse, that love is God. Perhaps that is the very move that can enable an acceptable gay theology. What would it be like to think of God as spirit--in particular, the spirit of resistance, as I have called it, manifest in the gay community, to think of God not as the spirit of God, but the spirit of resistance as God?

What would be gained by such a move? In the first instance, to recognize the spirit of resistance as God would be to acknowledge its compellingness and authoritativeness for us. To identify this variant of what we honorifically hail as the human spirit as god would be a way of recognizing that it is god for us, that it is appropriate for us to incarnate it. Indeed, one of the traditional functions of the term "God" is to name the focus of ultimate allegiance in the light of which all other allegiances are to be ordered. Moreover, in times of doubt and despair, we could thus recall ourselves to the sacrality of our vocation to embody the divine spirit of resistance. More can be said, but we must first explore the contours of this spirit that characterizes the gay community's engagement with AIDS.

First of all, this spirit takes offense, nay, is horrified at the violation, the disfigurement, the disablement, and the death which is AIDS--seeing this violation as desecration not merely of the bodies, but of the very selves of our friends and lovers. We are our bodies. It is by virtue of our embodiment that we are present in the world and the world is present to us. The defilement of our bodies is our defilement. The spirit of resistance is grounded in righteous anger that nature has visited us with this defilement and disruption of our lives and that our society has rested content with our individual, if not corporate, expendability. But anger passes over into compassion and resolve--the resolve, above all, that AIDS not have the last word, the resolve never to be in complicity with the destruction that is AIDS. We hope for the health of the infected, and until cure is a prospect, we hope for a life as rich as possible for the afflicted. We hope for a life free of the threat of AIDS, that there be life after AIDS for our whole community. And perhaps there is a hint of yet another hope. Robert Trent concludes a beautifully wistful article he wrote for *Christopher Street* entitled "Love and Death: Gay Sexuality in the Eighties" with the following:

> I know that gay is not love: to resist them--the ones that hate us--has always been part of it. Sometimes we are a delinquent peer group. We do not intend to keep dying. The nuclear family will not achieve that victory over us. I miss so many of you--living and dead. Even you that I hated unjustly because you had the nerve to say "No." I miss you and I hope we can get us back.
>
> In the midst of death is life. [17]

I should not want to press Trent too far. But if his hope "to get us back" is not merely a wish, but a hope--and if his hope is for each and every one, rather than just for our corporate life--then we can see the emergence of something like a hope for life after AIDS in even stronger terms, for it would include hope for life after AIDS even for the dead.

To think of God in terms of this complex of anger, resolve, and hope is not necessarily to reduce the reality of the divine to an aspect of human virtue. If we are called to hope, then we must think of spirit as active in more than the merely human. If our hopes are to be vindicated, we must allow some way by which evil may yet be overcome. As the existential philosopher Marcel argued, our hopes can be vindicated only if

...there is at the heart of being, beyond all data, beyond all inventories and all calculations, a mysterious principle which is in connivance with me, which cannot but will that which I will, if what I will deserves to be willed and is, in fact, willed by the whole of my being.[18]

Because our hopes outstrip what we can possibly (if we can hope for life after AIDS even for the dead) or probably (who can be fully spirited, spiritual in the sense in which I have developed it, all the time?) deliver, for the sake of our hope we can postulate a creativity in "connivance" with us. In my words, for the sake of our hope, we can imagine human spirit as characteristic of more than the human, and we can imagine it effective in ways other than through the human.

We should not think of divine spirit as *the* creative power which is *the* source of the universe, for the divine needs to be conceived by us only as pervasive and as powerful as would guarantee that our hopes not be vain. To be sure, God has traditionally been identified above all as "Creator" and philosophically defined variously as that without which we would not have being. In the traditional mythos, the Creator God is then discovered to be also the Redeemer God, that is, finally good. But what if "redeemer" is the basal metaphor, that is, that in virtue of which God is God? This would not mean that issues of power would then be irrelevant, but that they would become of second order. Indeed, one might very well hope that redemptive goodness could and would redeem all evil. In this way God could be understood as final power: to want to say that the Redeemer is also the Creator is really to hope that the Redeeming Power is finally powerful enough to effect a victory over everything in "creation." In this view, God's "creatorship" would be an eschatological, rather than an originative, function. If Redeemer, rather than Creator, names the ultimate role which makes divinity

divinity, then we can legitimately speak of a spirit in the world as God. If so, we can also speak of God in such a way as to avoid the intellectual bafflement of the problem of evil, for God, as the spirit of resistance, is in engagement with the world, rather than its ground or source.

Moreover, in imaging or understanding God as spirit, we are not thinking of God as a self. Spirit is a principal of inspiration, animation, vitalization of a self, but not a self itself. An athlete might show himself spirited by his show of "heart"--the spirit that he shows is not another self. It is a qualification of his selfhood. We can think of spirit in the ancient metaphor of "wind" rather than as a self.

Thus it seems to me that it is not illegitimate to speak of the "spirit of resistance" manifest in the fight of the gay community with AIDS as its god. First it is god because it is that which we as gays feel called upon to manifest it in our lives. But, secondly, it is our god because we hope. Fortunato has it wrong. We do not hope because we believe--rather we believe because we hope: the notion of divine spirit I am developing here, manifest in the human but more widely operative, is a postulate of hope. It need be envisioned only as large and as effective as the scope of that for which we hope, for ultimately to think of spirit in this way is a way of assuring us of the possibility of that for which we hope. Some would argue that the religious affirmation is ultimately reducible to the claim that the universe is on our side. Rather, religion, as envisioned here, claims something in the universe in alliance with human aspiration sufficiently large and powerful that humanity's hopes *might* prove justified. Religion confirms our identity, sanctioning what we are to become, and reassures us that our hopes are not doomed from the outset. I do not argue that good is our final destiny, only that the universe is constituted in such a way that it may be. ***God is the name for the reality of the possibility that there may yet be life after AIDS.***

To be sure, the fight against AIDS is not merely a life of uninterrupted battle. Whatever the case with individuals, the community still strives to play and to love--in however innovative ways. In Camus' novel *The Plague*, the only relief from the oppressive atmosphere of the plague comes when Dr. Rieux and Tarrou, the two central characters, go for a swim. It is an instructive incident. Within the novel, it serves to revive both for the characters and for the reader a sense of the integrity of life which the plague violates. So too, it is our play and our love play that keeps us in touch at a gut level with the reality which AIDS violates and in the name of which we protest and resist. No life, including religious life, can be unrelenting moral effort. I suggest that the spiritual, indeed the religious, life of the gay community exists finally in the rhythmic interplay between its play and the fight with AIDS. Ultimately the spirit of resistance is born from the frustration of worldly delight. The bodily delight which is the play of the gay community fires its life: it is that which AIDS frustrates and thus provokes the dissent which is the resistance to AIDS; and it defines the hope, the shape of the "life" for which we hope. In our soberer moments, we may be content to settle for more life for the living--and, in our more inspired moments, we dare aspire to more life even for the dead. But when we are most inspired, when we allow spirit to envision its own most ideal, it is then that the spirit of resistance reveals itself as spirit in search of a world to which it can give its unreserved assent, a world which is the sphere of unmitigated delight, not another world, but this world utterly transformed. What cannot be imagined may nevertheless be the object of hope, a world so utterly transformed that lions lie down with lambs and the dead overflow in bodily delight.

I have penned a credo for those who can see God through gay eyes:

I trust in
>   hold as sacred
>   hope to give myself over to

the spirit of self-abandon which
>   joys in life and rejoices in beauty,
>   in convivial solidarity with, and compassion for, all creatures,
>   and in the freedom to go out of my way for another.

I hope in the omnipotence of love,
>   that what love delights in will be established,
>   and what offends the heart of love will be overcome.

And I look for the transfiguration of all flesh in unambiguous life.

In our fight with AIDS, we want a fighting chance. "God" as I have used the term is the name of that reality by which our struggle may not prove an eternal defeat, and our hopes may not be in vain. *If* hope for life after AIDS is really but a cipher for a hope for life and more life, life abundant even for the dead, then we can give our lives and give up our dead in hope.

How wide an appeal such a religious view might have I cannot speculate. I do think that it makes contact with other spiritual movements of our day, the protests of the civil rights era, and the "never again" of the Holocaust and Hiroshima survivors. Whether such a vision is specifically Christian could be argued. But a person could do worse than choosing such a credo to live by. To echo Unamuno, if death is our ultimate destiny, living out such a credo would make of our deaths an injustice.[19]

---

[1]To date, I have been unable to relocate the source for this statement.

[2]John J. McNeill, *The church and the homosexual.* Third Edition, Updated and Expanded (Boston: Beacon, 1988) and *Taking a chance on God: Liberating theology for gays, lesbians, and their lovers, families, and friends* (Boston: Beacon, 1989).

[3]John E. Fortunato, *Embracing the exile: Healing journeys of gay Christians* (San Francisco: Harper & Row, 1982) and *AIDS, the spiritual dilemma* (San Francisco: Harper & Row, 1987).

[4]For the text and discussion, see Jeannine Grammick and Pat Furey, eds., *The Vatican and homosexuality: Reactions to the "Letter to the bishops of the Catholic Church on the pastoral care of homosexual persons"* (New York: Crossroads, 1988).

[5]*Ibid.,* pp. 207-215.

[6]*Ibid.,* p. 207.

[7]This is the approach taken by gay theologian J. Michael Clark. See his *A place to start: Toward an unapologetic gay liberation theology* (Dallas: Monument Press, 1989), pp. 65-78, and the essay "AIDS, suffering and theology" in his *Gay being, divine presence: Essays in gay spirituality* (Garland: Tangelwuld Press, 1987), pp. 55-75. However, in opting for a "process" theodicy (*i.e.,* God is not omnipotent), it seems to me that Clark compromises what I have long thought the genius of the Western tradition, the right to be in a lover's quarrel with the world order, the natural as well as the sociopolitical and economic orders. And it is this dimension of the tradition that I find crucial in the development of a timely gay theology. I take up process theodicy in more detail in my rejoinder to Clark in this volume.

[8]Fortunato, *AIDS, op cit.*

[9]*Ibid.,* pp. 94ff.

[10]*Ibid.,* p. 85.

[11]Albert Camus, *The plague.* Trans. by Stuart Gilbert (New York: Vintage, 1972).

[12]McNeill, *Taking a chance on God, op cit.,* p. 14.

[13]This line of thought follows Gordon Kaufman's distinction between the *real* and the *available* referent for the idea of God as developed in *God the problem* (Cambridge, MA: Harvard University, 1972), pp. 84 ff.

[14]*Cf.,* for example, Emmanuel Dreuilhe, *Mortal Embrace: Living with AIDS.* Trans. by Linda Coverdale (New York: Hill and Wang, 1988) and Paul Monette, *Borrowed time: An AIDS memoir* (New York: Harcourt, Brace, Manovich, 1988).

[15]Albert Camus, *The rebel: An essay in revolt.* Trans. by Anthony Bower (New York: Vintage, 1956).

[16]Ruben Alves, *What is religion?* (Maryknoll, NY: Orbis, 1981), p. 88.

[17]*Christopher Street* (Issue 116). Vol. 10, No. 8 (New York: That New Magazine), p. 31.

[18]Gabriel Marcel, "On the ontological mystery," quoted in James L. Muyskens, *The sufficiency of hope: The conceptual foundations of religion* (Philadelphia: Temple University, 1979), p. 86. The entire work of Muyskens is relevant to my approach to religious reality, as is the work of Fontinell. See Eugene Fontinell, *Toward a reconstruction of religion* (West Nyack, NY: Cross Currents, 1970) and the more recent *Self, God, and immortality: A Jamesian investigation* (Philadelphia: Temple University, 1986).

[19]Miguel de Unamuno, *The tragic sense of life in men and nations*. Trans. by Anthony Kerrigan (Princeton University/Bollingen Series, 1972), p. 286. Unamuno here is actually adapting a quote from Sénancour.

II. Gay Vision & Constructive Theology:
A Response
J. Michael Clark, PH.D.

Without our identities being known to either of us at the time, I originally encountered Ron Long's work in an earlier draft, when I was called upon to review his essay for the Fourth Annual Lesbian, Bisexual, and Gay Studies Conference held at Harvard in October 1990. In retrospect I have realized that, partially given my own professional quandary and sense of isolation at the time, many of my comments were either too picayune or too personal. Nonetheless, the revised final version of "God through Gay Men's Eyes" is both a tribute to Dr. Long and, even more importantly, an invaluable contribution to the small but growing dialogue which is developing constructive and unapologetically pro-gay/lesbian liberation theology. And, while he has acknowledged in our more recent correspondence--and gladly so--that we have "variant perspectives" on certain issues, I think we both agree in desiring to celebrate and (re)affirm the diversity of *all* our voices in this emerging dialogue. It is in just this spirit that I offer my response to his work here, in the hope of further nurturing theological and spiritual explorations throughout our varied community.

One of the many valuable services Long's essay performs is to provide a critical perspective on the work of John J. McNeill and John E. Fortunato,[1] particularly in regard to theologizing for the AIDS health crisis era in our community. McNeill's failure to pursue the consequences of AIDS for theology and Fortunato's failure to resolve the issue of theodicy (god/ess' omnipotence) are not in fact the best resources we have on these issues. Specifically, for example, Fortunato fails intellectually on two counts: Admitting "bafflement" and resorting to a Koan are very poor alternatives to rigorously considering sounder alternatives to theodicy (the problem of evil) such as those represented in process thought and elsewhere. Moreover, the Jobian "right to be in a lover's quarrel with the world order" and/or with god/ess keeps the faithful in an argumentative mode and does nothing to facilitate action. Realizing the limitations, and sometimes even the impotence, of the divine forces *people* to (re)assume responsibility(ies) for action--both justice-making and care-giving.

Related to this concern is another important strength in Long's work--his recognition that "classical theism" provides very little constructive help for those of us dealing with AIDS. I especially like his comment that "it strains credibility ... to suppose that a god who would send AIDS could be trusted to provide a future even for the dead"; although I may be somewhat unclear about the *exact* way in which Long himself resolves theodicy, I do applaud the implications at least of his metaphor of resistance for this problem. Connecting theodicy with this metaphor and reconceptualizing God *in godself* as resistance is very intriging. God as resistance and hope (as horizontal, present and futureward energies), rather than as vertical creator and ground, eliminates altogether making the divine in any way responsible for AIDS. God as resistance also entails the ethical demand that we "incarnationally" join in "radical participation" in healing and care-giving, as well as across the full range of liberation-seeking, sociopolitical activities.[2] Even our love-making exudes a fecundity which nurtures the divine-as-resistance into fuller being!

The strongest point in Long's work may in fact be his elaboration of the metaphor of resistance as a key concept for reconstructing theology from a gay/lesbian perspective. As gay men and lesbians collectively resist ho-

mophobia (human evil) and AIDS (natural evil), we become a corporate incarnation of, or a community of, resistance; that is a very powerful liberation theology motif.
Sharon Welch's work, as well as the great bulk of Latin
American liberation theology, provide the necessary prece-
dents for further grounding this very significant metaphor.[3]

Yet another related point of importance is Long's
affirmation of radical embodiment and anger, both as theological motifs in their own right and also as part and parcel
of "resistance." Our embodied anger at AIDS--at its dev-
astation of our community and specifically at its devasta-
tion of the bodies of our friends and lovers, as well as at sociopolitical failures to adequately respond to the crisis--is
the motivating and, I would say, divinely inspired and nur-
tured energy which fuels our resistance, our liberational efforts. Similarly, one of gay/lesbian theology's strenths is its
ability to (re)unite spirituality and sexuality. Not only have
contemporary gayspirit writers addressed this,[4] but so do
Fortunato and the Catholic heritage (e.g., twelfth century
St. Aelred of Rievaulx[5]).

One caveat, however: The exclusion of a thoroughgoing consideration of the feminist and/or lesbian/feminist
theological canon here means that Long does not articulate
the supportive detail for pursuing the (re)valuation of experience and bodiliness for liberation theology to the extent
which lesbian/feminists already have. Because established
feminist analyses and categories are so closely related to
gay/lesbian concerns already, ignoring their work risks
placing Long in the position of "reinventing the wheel."
Nevertheless, his radical affirmation that *we are our bodies*
implicitly resonates with the insights of our lesbian/femi-
nist colleagues.

Finally, some of the nicest portions of the essay,
from the standpoint of artistic and interdisciplinary craft,
are those in which Long compares Camus' fictional work
with the real AIDS crisis and its theological implications--

an obvious, to me at least, comparison which I have long wished someone would undertake in depth. While it might, however, be more poignant to pull all of the Camus references and discussion into one location, as they stand these comments work like a recurring counterpoint to weave together a singular and fine composition. In short, it is most encouraging to find Ron Long's voice joining the small but growing chorus of gay men and lesbians who are unabashedly seeking liberation through the (re)construction of theology.

---

[1]John J. McNeill, *Taking a chance on God: Liberating theology for gays, lesbians, their lovers, families, and friends* (Boston: Beacon, 1988); John E. Fortunato, *AIDS, the spiritual dilemma* (San Francisco: Harper & Row, 1987).

[2]cf., I. Carter Heyward, *Our passion for justice: Images of power, sexuality, and liberation* (New York: Pilgrim, 1984).

[3]Sharon D. Welch, "Ideology and social change," *Weaving the visions: New patterns in feminist spirituality* (J. Plaskow & C.P. Christ, eds.; San Francisco: Harper & Row, 1989), pp. 336-343; Thomas M. Thurston, "Gay theology of liberation and the hermeneutic circle," *Constructing gay theology* (M.L. Stemmeler & J.M. Clark, eds.; Dallas: Monument, 1991), pp. 7-26, and *Gay theology of liberation*, unpublished manuscript.

[4]Mark Thompson (ed.), *Gay spirit: Myth and meaning* (New York: St. Martins, 1987).

[5]J. Michael Clark, *Gay being, divine presence: Essays in gay spirituality* (Garland, TX: Tangelwüld, 1987), pp. 48-54.

III. Revisioning & Renewing:
A Rejoinder
Ronald E. Long, PH.D.

I remember my excitement when I discovered the writings of J. Michael Clark and the profound pleasure I took in reading them. Although it had taken me years to realize how deeply my own theological reflections had been informed by my experience as a gay man and to begin self-consciously to employ my gayness as a theological starting point, here was a man who was already writing and publishing on fundamental theological issues from an un-apologetic gay perspective. The meeting with the man himself was a source of yet further delight. Having just shaken hands at the convention of the American Academy of Religion in New Orleans in November 1990, he was already graciously eager to read my own efforts. Further communication has only confirmed what I had hoped for, that in him I had encountered a colleague! Now I am honored, both personally and professionally, that Clark should write a response to my essay and volunteer that our work appear together as a dialogue. Clark's written response, here offered publicly, represents a formal welcome into the incipient dialogue which is gay theology. Mutual public recognition is important for those of us who are, in essence, creating a new discipline. Beyond that, however, both Clark and I agree that gay theology is work that needs to be done. Naming god and naming ourselves are mutually implied acts that ought to be pursued self-consciously, with real attention to our specific situation as gay men in the age of AIDS. We both hope to provoke a wider discussion yet, and our joint offering here is a symbol of our desire for ongoing dialogue. We are confident that such a theological enterprise will prove of service in the cause of gay liberation and the further development of the modern understanding of God.

One of the great contributions of feminist theory has been its challenge to the notion that any one person or community can speak for all. Our insights are inherently perspectival, and thus limited. I cannot help but speak as a man and as a gay man at that. To pretend to do otherwise is as pretentious as it is impossible in fact. If I cannot speak from a universal perspective, then theology must be an act of confessional self-clarification: "This is how it stands with me." And thus begins a dialogue: "How stands it with you? What should each of us think in the light of our mutual confessions?"[1] Such a dialogue is an opportunity for self-clarification and refinement--and dialogue thus becomes theology's refining fire. But that is to touch upon yet another theme of feminist thinking and theo/thealogy, namely the thoroughgoing construction of the self in its interrelating.

Clark chides me for my inattention in my essay to currents in feminist theology. To fail to make the connections, and thereby marshall support in our battle with homophobia and heterosexism, is indeed a political blunder at this point. But Clark seems to imply that my failure to invoke feminist writers puts me in a position of having to "reinvent the wheel." His phrasing suggests that one can take feminist thinking on embodiment as a *fait accompli* and build from there. Ironically, the essay to which he refers endorses the pedagogic value of "reinventing the wheel."[2] I would submit moreover that theology, in particular, is an enterprise that proceeds and renews itself only as it rethinks and reappropriates--reinvents--its heritage from the ground up. However that may be, feminist thinking on embodiment itself can be seen as a reworking of the existential idea of "being in a situation" and, insofar as embodiment

implies situatedness (social, biological, and ecological)--
being "matrixed"--an appropriation of the claim of process
philosophers that, ontologically speaking, being-in-relation
is the basal structure of all existence. And Whitehead himself, the father of process philosophy, spoke of his own efforts as a "transformation of some main doctrines of Absolute Idealism on to a realistic basis," noting moreover of
Process and Reality that "though throughout the main body
of the work I am in sharp disagreement with Bradley, the
final outcome is after all not so greatly different."[3] To me,
some of the inadequacies of idealism continue to haunt
both its feminist and process successors. And, while I am
certain that all authentic theology is "reinvention," I am
even more convinced that unapologetic gay theology in our
day, in the age of AIDS, should not simply assume any position from any tradition unqualifiedly and should dare to
chart its own independent course.

Clark rightly senses the importance of Camus in the
development of my own thought. I think it is to Camus'
credit that he strove to be sensitive to the ways in which we
make treaties with evil--or, in the language of *The Rebel*
and *The Plague,* the ways in which we justify murder. We
adopt systems of thought, positions which rationalize, and
thus render acceptable, what on a gut level is but unaccept-
able. Sacrifice of something or someone becomes morally
acceptable when demanded by the good of the group or the
future or the system...or whatever. For Camus, to embrace
any such "system" is to compromise our horror at the sacrifice which the system "requires." And that is ultimately to
dilute our sense of the evilness of evil and undermine our
efforts to combat it.

A similar concern for the integrity of our notions of
good and evil animated George Santayana's criticism of the
idealism of Josiah Royce. The idea of the thoroughgoing
social construction of the self, the self as a dialogic reality,
had been brilliantly developed in Royce. Axiomatic for

him, moreover, was the idea that self-affirmation implied endorsement of whatever group or system in virtue of which the self was constituted as an individual. Santayana rightly perceived difficulty here:

> Royce never recoiled from a paradox or a bitter fact: and he used to say that a mouse, when tormented and torn to pieces by a cat, was realizing his own deepest will, since he had subconsciously chosen to be a mouse in a world that should have cats in it. The mouse, really, in his deeper self, wanted to be terrified, clawed, and devoured.[4]

To be sure, Santayana's reportage here tends to ride roughshod over important subtleties in Royce's published writings. But what Santayana rightly sensed was Royce's failure to give sufficient credence to the difference between the moral interests of the creature and the demands and necessities of the system of which s/he may be a part.

Santayana himself, attempting to avoid what he called the moral error of pantheism, was led to draw an important distinction between "worship" and "piety." Piety, for Santayana, was "man's reverent attachment to the sources of his being and the steadying of his life by that attachment."[5] Whereas worship involves the attribution of unambiguous worth, piety entails an honoring which is compatible with the acknowledgement of fault in the revered object. Thus the universe, the system of nature, could be an object of piety without being an appropriate object of worship:

> The universe is the true Adam, the creation of the true fall; and as we have never blamed our mythical first parent very much, in spite of the disproportionate consequences of his sin because we felt that he was but human and that we, in his place, might have sinned too, so we may easily forgive our real ancestor, whose connatural sin we are from moment to

moment committing, since it is only the necessary rashness of
venturing to be without foreknowing the price or fruits of existence.[6]

I have always thought Santayana's distinction a wise one.
But it is a subtlety which is lost in any system which images the world of nature as "god/dess' body"--or our primordial "matrix" as an aspect of god/dess' being--as much
feminist "thealogy" does.[7]

A distinguishable, but frequently complementary,
position is that worked out in the tradition of process philosophy, where God is pictured as ultimately responsible for
the existence of evil, but is not blameworthy on that account. Rather than picture God as omnipotent, omniscient,
and all-good, process theodicists image deity as limited in
power: some aspects of creation are out of divine hands
and are to be understood as necessary aspects of created
being. While God may be responsible for evil in the world
because the world in fact exists only because of divine creativity, God is not blameworthy, because any evils that exist as part of the world are inescapably a potential aspect of
material being which is otherwise good. The claim is that
the world would have to be something as we know it if
there is to be any world at all. While I do think it episte-
mologically presumptuous to dare to think that our kind of
world is the only really possible kind, I am more concerned
with the way in which certain evils--the so-called "natural"
evils, in particular--now become acceptable as the "cost" of
creation. The evils to which flesh is vulnerable are now
justified as the acceptable price of God's "good" creation.
Such a theology can hardly be good news to the afflicted:
"You may be sick and dying--but, unless we were vulnerable to sickness, no one could enjoy existence." But then
the happiness of the currently healthy seems to be purchased at the cost of the suffering and expendability of the
afflicted.

To be sure, process thinkers couple such an understanding of creation with a doctrine of God as the pre-eminently sensitive one, the co-experiencer of all things. And in experiencing our experience, God appreciates our efforts, our joys, and our pains. God thus emerges as the comforting friend in our pain. Since God is also eternal, at no time are our losses unappreciated; God's memory spares our personal tragedies from having made no difference to anyone and thus from final insignificance. But note clearly, it is our lives, not our persons, that God thus saves. And note further, this is the same God who finds our personal tragedies the "acceptable" price of creation. Such a view asks the sick to see themselves as the unlucky victims where the ills that flesh is prone to are exemplified. And to the extent illness is terminal, it asks the sick to see their untimely expendability as one of the costs of existence elected by God in his eagerness to create.[8] How much of a sympathetic ally does God appear in such a light? Better to stop thinking of God as creator, the origin of all things, than to see Him/Her as the one who elects me to live only to suffer and to die. Theodicy is an impossible game, and God must be totally reconceived if belief in God is ever to be morally credible.

In his response to my essay, however, Clark does raise a terribly important issue. While commending me for using "resistance" as a metaphor for divine and faithful life, he does wonder if such a stance does not make one too "argumentative." I am reminded of a parallel criticism of Camus in the work of Marcel.[9] While recognizing Camus' concern to avoid any system or faith that compromises our sensitivity to and therefore responsiveness to evil, Marcel wonders whether the stance of "revolt" does not itself prove compromising, in certain circumstances at least. Camus feared that hope would be hope either for an act of deliverance by another that would render the self's efforts obsolete or for a future good that could be purchased only by the present evil. In the first instance, action becomes unnecessary. In the second, the sense of the vileness of evil--the stimulus for action--is undercut. Marcel, on the other hand, argued that certain forms of resignation and refusal to hope blind the self to the potentialities for action within a given situation: it is hope that frees the self up enough so that the self has the space to sense opportunity. He thus invokes the image of the war resister, hoping for the downfall of the occupying force, rather than that of Camus' *l'homme revolté* as morally compelling. And if one can think that not every good that comes out of evil thereby justifies that evil, then it would seem that Marcel has the more compelling position here. Thus I have striven to envision the divine spirit as both resistant and hopeful, and the life of faith as the rhythmic interplay between affirmation and resistance.

The issue for Clark and myself, as for Camus and Marcel, has to do with the integrity of life, with conceptual adequacy in picturing life, and with the consequent success in grounding our values and life-stance. Clark has challenged me on the grounds that my way of thinking of God and faith seems to lead to an "argumentative" stance which compromises the potentiality for fullness of life. So too, I have been arguing that feminist theology and process theodicy are inadequate propadeutic instruments for gay theology because, as they stand now, they compromise our sense of the evilness of evil and thus our engagement with it. Thus, Clark continues to struggle with the notion of a God who is somehow a personal being, while I am led to envision a spirit which is not the spirit of an otherwise existent reality called God. But, if both Clark and I seem really concerned about the attitudes and stances which our positions tend to elicit and foster, we would appear to have uncovered grounds for judging the success of our respective speculative programs: does this position really foster this particular life-stance? is this particular stance a truly humane one? However, an alternative assessment of the situation looms over the horizon.

Fackenheim's work has successfully demonstrated the dialectical character of rabbinic theology.[10] Over and over again the rabbis of tradition found themselves affirming mutually exclusive and often contradictory ideas: for example, God is at once in control but is, at the same time, solicitous of human "obedience." So too, Fackenheim himself discerns the commanding Voice of Auschwitz which, in seeking to deny Hitler a posthumous victory, bids the religious Jew to be religious in revolutionarily new ways-- while it bids the secular Jew not to let the Jewish faith disappear as a factor in Jewish life. Individual concepts are inadequate to do justice to reality, much less divine reality. For Fackenheim, then, religious thought and practice are opened up by the space generated by contradictory affirmations. And perhaps gay theology should rightly understand itself at this time as equally dialectical.

It is true that we need each other to come to full self-consciousness. To echo a Roycean quip, how do I know what I think until I have been challenged to formulate it? We need each other as midwives to our individual thoughts. Dialogue might be justified on these grounds alone. But what if theology, and gay theology in particular, must be carried on dialectically? Perhaps religious reality-- and religious living--only opens up to view in the interaction of our respective speculative commitments. I have often described the study of religion to my students at Hunter College as a matter of empathetically exploring many different traditions and points of view until one begins to develop a "taste" for religion. Perhaps the success of our theologizing is the taste for reality opened up by the dialogue among the theologians *and* the interaction of their theologies. To invoke another metaphor, perhaps our respective speculative and systematic allegiances are but guideposts which map out a given territory. If that is true, then it is highly important that the nascent theological discussion of our community blossom. And it is with pride that I offer my reflections in dialogue with J. Michael Clark in the hope that a dialogue that will serve the liberation of our community may flourish.

---

[1]This formulation derives from N. Morton. *Cf.* J. Michael Clark, *A Place to start: Toward an unapologetic gay liberation theology* (Dallas: Monument Press, 1989), p. 5.

[2]Sharon Welch, "Ideology and social change" in Judith Plaskow and Carol P. Christ, eds., *Weaving the visions: New patterns in feminist spirituality* (San Francisco: Harper & Row, 1989), pp. 337f.

[3]Quoted in Frederick Copleston, S.J., *A history of philosophy. Vol. VIII: Bentham to Russell* (Westminster, MD: The Newman Press, 1966), pp. 399f.

[4]George Santayana, *Character and opinion in the United States* (New York: Norton, 1967), p. 115.

[5]George Santayana, *Reason in religion* (New York, Dover, 1982), p. 179.

[6]*Ibid.*, p. 192.

[7]For the former, see Rosemary Radford Ruether, *Sexism & Godtalk: Toward a feminist theology* (Boston: Beacon, 1983) and Sallie McFague, *Models of God: Theology for an ecological, nuclear age* (Philadelphia: Fortress, 1987). Carter Heyward's otherwise admirable theology stands as an example of the latter. For her, God is to be imaged in three ways: "God is our relational matrix (or womb). God is born in our relational matrix. God is becoming our relational matrix." *Touching our strength: The erotic as power and the love of God* (San Francisco: Harper & Row, 1989), p. 23.

[8]It might be argued, of course, that creation does not take place by choice: God's nature is to be creative. However, it seems to me that if one wanted to preserve the idea that God creates out of love, one would have to allow for the metaphor of choice. To the extent that God creates merely because God's nature is to be creative, God's nature as sympathetic friend is compromised. In this latter case, the shade of Voltaire can be heard in the background: what need have we of such a hypothesis?

[9]Here it is instructive to compare Marcel's characterization of hope in his essay "Sketch of a phenomenology and a metaphysic of hope" (*Homo viator: Introduction to a metaphysic of hope.* Trans. by Emma

Crauford [Harper & Row, 1962], pp. 37ff.) with his critique of Camus in "The refusal of salvation and the exaltation of the man of absurdity" in the same volume (pp. 200 ff.)

[10]Emil Fackenheim, *God's presence in history* (San Francisco: Harper & Row, 1972), esp. p. 1.

IV. Toward a Lavender Credo:
From Theology to Belief
J. Michael Clark, Ph.D.

In memory of **Gary Picola, Robert Needle, Serge Bernstein,** and all the others. And with deep appreciation to Congregation Bet Haverim, Atlanta.

I am possessed by god/ess--by muses and eros--pursued by Ganymede, infused by Dionysus, lured by Pan. I am obsessed with the pluriform Oneness, the Mysteriousness which defies metaphors and names. The gentleness of dawn, the passion of love-making, the poignancy of co-suffering, the silence of evening. Theologizing is a never-ending, never-completing, ever-weaving, dialogical process toward wholeness: finding and hearing, speaking and listening, our voices bespeaking god/ess, our lives yearning toward our fullest liberation and in the yearning creating--by speaking, writing, acting--that very liberation. Still, nearly a decade postdoctoral, as many books as years spun forth in the weaving, I am still obsessed with that which possesses me--theophile, god/ess-lover in all the pluriform manifestations of godself's mysterious disclosures. I cannot *not* think, respond, and write of that weaving web of meaningfulness. And, so, I begin again, revisiting my starting places,[1] revisioning my own visions, simplifying and realizing what I really believe--in this fragmentary instant: *Credo!*

As my dialogue with Ron Long has again reminded me, the activity of doing theology is, indeed, a fragmentary and ongoing process. As a dialogue between experience and tradition which emphasizes the prophetic strand of our two-pronged Judaeo-Christian tradition in opposition to any oppressive or exclusionary strands in that same tradition, gay liberation theology in particular is simultaneously the search for and the realization of each individual's own voice. As such, and as the late Nelle Morton has reminded us, it remains always both confessional and invitational: "This is how it is with me. How is it with you?"[2] It is also a radical (re)assertion of our lives as *the* authoritative source for theology. All texts, all dogmas, and all creeds are subjected to this criterion: If they do not liberate, they do not embody god/ess' energy. Consequently, our gay/lesbian liberational spirituality--our theological activity--*is* political action of a radical sort. As are, of course, our very lives! These caveats remain my theological methodology. Indeed, the urgency toward liberation inherent in my approach to theology-as-activity, further discloses itself in the pluriform rationale which necessitates continuing the process, the dialogue, still so young and frail, which those of us doing gay liberation theology must continue to nurture.

Among the ongoing rationale for continuing to pursue gay liberation theology, as well as to seek yet other, more accessible ways to express--to give voice to--this theological activity, remains our own continued awareness as lesbians and gay men of our difference within a heterosexist, patriarchally constructed society. Homophobia, sodomy laws, the lack of legal protections for our coupled relationships, discrimination in hiring practices, obstacles to professional fulfillment--altogether these manifestations and structures of heterosexism and patriarchy demand a continuing prophetic voice announcing god/ess with and for us. Moreover, apologetic efforts in both biblical studies, pastoral theology, and denominational politics are still futile dead ends, even when offered with the most compassionate of intentions.[3] The majoritarian structure of our democratic institutional religious forms remain heteropatriarchal.

One other rationale is also worth reiterating: As an ongoing process, gay liberation theology must continue to assert and to reassert an adamant reaffirmation that being gay or lesbian is not just about sex.[4] Indeed, as I have said in a slightly different way elsewhere, most of us who are gay or lesbian have come to realize that being gay is far more than just a matter of sexual behavior; it is rather a whole mode of being-in-the world, an existential standpoint which colors all our perceptions of and interactions with the world and one which also stands over against established cultural and religious standards for gender roles and intimate human relationships.[5]

And so, I again take up the task of exploring belief, of doing theology. And, of claiming my own voice, of invoking dialogue. My way back into this dialogue is through the vehicle of another. Rereading the complete corpus of novelist Chaim Potok re-confronted me with my place between and beyond the prongs of our inherited western tradition. His voice created a mirror for appraising my own. As a result, I have been led to re-examine my intellectual efforts to develop a complete and thoroughgoing gay liberation theology. The seeming wholeness--complete--of scholarly activity belies the fragmentary, processive nature of theology-as-activity. Liberation theology is fluid, changing, and so no one effort to insert oneself into this fluidity can ever be final. Moreover, the thoroughgoingness of scholarly work can also veil the real simplicity and accessibility of liberational faith. Potok's vehicle has cast me back upon the shores of intellectual curiosity with a new tool--lenses not of academic achievement or of professional aspiration, but of community and relationship. My spouse's own caveat to "keep it simple" has at last penetrated my psyche and I am able to begin to peel back the layers of academese to see what is really there, what is really worth sharing, what is really worth voicing as invitation.

My immersion in Potok's Jewish faith community and my own claiming theological activity as believing, as "faithing," have also led me to reconsider elements not fully pursued in my work to date--where I stand as a gay liberation theologian in relation to religious holidays, rituals, and even prayer--strange concerns perhaps for an ardently anti-institutional theologian such as myself, but something which I can no longer ignore. Having thus attempted to simplify the activity of theology--for myself as well as for those who share their voices with mine in the dialogue--and having completed a portion of my own unfinished business, I will attempt to weave these strands together to (re)create my own particular voice. Richard Rubenstein has insisted that "all theologies are inherently subjective. ... The theologian ... is in reality communicating an inner world [he/she] suspects others may share."[6] My efforts here remind me again of his insight and so I offer these thoughts to you, gentle reader, knowing full well they must of necessity remain fragmentary, incomplete, everchanging--my own confessional voice, empassioned by a divine obsession, joining other voices. Let yours also be heard.

(i) Religious Identity & the Writing of Chaim Potok

I first encountered the novels and historical writing of Chaim Potok[7] when, as a non-Jew with a growing belief in monotheism and an ardent curiosity about Judaism, I found myself the alchemical agent bringing together two Jews so that the three of us could start a gay and lesbian synagogue. My then best friend has since died of AIDS and my now ex-lover has long since found elements in the sexual subculture more powerful in their attraction for him than his native Judaism. Nor am I, the *goyische* cofounder, any longer affiliated with the synagogue. Fortunately, however, more than six years after its founding,

Congregation Bet Haverim remains a vital and growing institution, ironically the only Reconstructionist synagogue in the Atlanta area.

Back then, I first read Potok to quench my thirst for an understanding of American Jewry in this century. I worked diligently for and faithfully attended our fledgling synagogue as I learned about Judaism both in worship and in Potok's fiction. Then, as I lost first my primary relationship and then my good friend, I no longer had a translator, an interpreter. The Hebrew began to seem too difficult again, the ethnicity too foreign for this southern-bred, formerly ordained, Methodist minister. The synagogue's subsequent collective decision to affiliate with the Reconstructionist and not the Reform movement (denomination) meant an enhanced focus not upon theology but upon ethnicity--an understandable need for isolated and heretofore estranged gay and lesbian Jews in the Protestant, heterosexual south. But now, I really was the outsider; I slipped out unnoticed one Friday night and have not returned.

That hungering for things theologically and symbolically associated with liberal Judaism did not abate, however. I whisper "good Shabbos" to god/ess and myself on Friday afternoons. I light Chanukah candles, embarrassedly mumbling my southern, accent-crippled Hebrew. I cherish Pesach (Passover) as an event symbolic, too, of my own liberation as a gay man--though I have no group with whom to share the Seder. I honor Yom HaShoah, remembering the Holocaust of six million Jews and a quarter million gay men. With Yom Kippur/Kol Nidre, I struggle with the seemingly bad theology of predestination in the age of AIDS, while I am nonetheless glad for the activity of remembering the ever-growing list of those whom we have lost. I very much want *Kaddish* (the traditional prayer for the dead) said for me when the time comes and I fear that I might have no one who will know to do that for me. And I avoid Israeli politics because I am a product of the separation of religion and government. Neither a post-Holocaust empathy for Judaism as a people, nor a theology influenced by Judaism as a religion, implies for me that the 20th century nation state of Israel is always right. Zionists, of course, will strongly disagree. Most Jews will dismiss me as a *goy*, anyway.

For Jews I must no doubt appear a *goyische* theologian; for the Christian *goyim* I may appear somewhat Jewish, but certainly not Christian. For both Jews and Christians, I am adamantly gay, and therefore easily dismissed by both groups. This particular gay liberation theologian still finds no institutional affiliation wherein to find a home and, since for the most part the gay/lesbian community remains distrustful of religion, I am left as it were to my own theological devices. My spouse of some three years now--raised Missouri Synod Lutheran, attracted and then repulsed by Pentecostalism during his army days--provides an empathetic, quasi new age support for my quandaries and explorations. He patiently reads all my manuscripts, lovingly making suggestions for revisions and clarity and, in one case, even more actively contributed to the writing of a book.[8] He is definitely good for me--spiritually, theologically, and otherwise. And yet, the hungering remains.

So, I have recently returned to Chaim Potok and reread all his novels. My meditations upon them are a part of my own struggle with religious identity, particularly as to whether I should remain an affiliational outsider. After all, the religious and theological margins have been my surest home for quite some time now. Potok's corpus seems a good companion for my dilemma, insofar as his novels show from different angles, like the facets of a single jewel, the conflict of love for one's religious tradition and a far-ranging quest for truths which are far less rigid than those of the tradition in its most orthodox forms. Throughout his books runs a passion for the religious Jewish tradition and its people, alongside his characters' efforts to create healthy bridges between pre-Holocaust, eastern European, orthodox (even Hasidic) Judaism and modern, post-Holocaust scholarship and belief.

Most striking are the extent to which the novels draw upon autobiography and the fact that the chronology by which they were written, or at least published, does not coincide with the internal chronology of the books themselves. Potok's sixth book, for example, *Davita's Harp*, covers approximately 1928-1942. Its foreground concerns non-religious, even communist-identified, Jews and non-Jews, specifically in regard to the Spanish Civil war. Simultaneously, Potok unravels his first-person heroine's quest--a child with no religious upbringing who is exposed to both Judaism, Christianity, and Communism--as she tries to discover and claim her own Jewish identity. As the novel moves toward its Jewish-affirmative ending, a significant subplot also unfolds. Davita is a strong, intelligent young woman who is denied public recognition for her achievement and who must come to claim her achievement only from within. She must learn that although she has been denied as a woman in a patriarchal religious environment, she herself will never forget. Those in power may be able to deny, but they cannot take away one's inner knowledge of accomplishment. The element of chronology emerges in these closing pages wherein Davita's only apparent champion among her peers is pre-Bar Mitzvah Reuven Malter, the narrator of Potok's first two novels.

In Potok's first novel, *The Chosen*, Reuven is fifteen, about two years after graduating from the yeshiva grammar school with Davita. It is 1944, just before D-Day. Young Danny Saunders is also introduced in this novel, along with his Rebbe father and the latter's problematic child-rearing method--Silence. Here, in his first novel, Potok sets up the struggle between an eastern Jewish, Hasidic orthodox tradition and the demands of post-Holocaust modernity, as an otherwise very religious young Hasid

(Danny) chooses to abdicate the hereditary tzaddikate (priesthood) to his sickly younger brother, in order to pursue a career in psychoanalysis. As the conflict between Freud and Talmud develops, Danny becomes an embodiment of the struggle to keep both elements balanced within one individual soul.

The second novel, *The Promise,* picks up this narrative almost immediately, elaborating the struggle between eastern European Hasidic orthodoxy and orthodox Judaism in the U.S. What appears as the burgeoning of Reconstructionism and/or secular Judaism threatens orthodoxy, particularly as textual biblical criticism is pitted against "revealed scriptures." Potok now discloses a wider variety of approaches to the difficulty of building bridges, particularly the contrast of insanity and successful integration. The adolescent son of the "reconstructionist" textual critic is almost destroyed by the conflict; interestingly, a now older Danny Saunders develops Silence as an effective, albeit desperate, mode of therapy for the young man. Because of the textual criticism conflict, Reuven's father must make a career change and Reuven himself is almost denied *smicha,* or ordination, from his orthodox school. What emerges most passionately in the character of Reuven is a healthy love of tradition. Reuven learns that he can in fact nurture, not destroy, the tradition with his scholarship, rather than by a fearful clinging to rigid old ideas.

To my reading there are some minor problems in the ways in which these two novels connect. In *The Chosen,* Danny's brother is very sickly, but in *The Promise* he is now simply the assumed heir to the father's role as tzaddik. Likewise, in *The Chosen* Reuven's father suffers two heart attacks, but in *The Promise* he is not only strong enough to complete his controversial book on scientific textual criticism, but is also strong enough to weather the ensuing controversy, to engage in numerous Zionist activities, and to relinquish his previous yeshiva position for a professorship in the liberal seminary. Even in the *The Chosen*, I am not clear why if Danny and Reuven started out in the same school level, and both are such brilliant students, that Reuven's ordination, central to *The Promise*, is a year after Danny's. Could that in some way reflect differences between Hasidism and orthodoxy which I know nothing about?

Potok's fourth novel, *In the Beginning,* overlaps the chronology of *Davita's Harp*, while focusing solely upon religious Jews. The main plot describes bringing eastern European Jews to America before Hitler makes that impossible. The Holocaust and the loss of family are important as secondary themes and, again, Potok's narrator, now David Lurie, chooses to strengthen the tradition of Talmudic scholarship by learning and using *goyische* textual criticism. This is also a heavily autobiographical novel, insofar as David's father, Max Lurie, is a combination of Potok's own father and father-in-law. Likewise, David's mother, who was nearly raped in a pogrom and who lost her betrothed to another pogrom, is drawn from Potok's mother. She was betrothed to Max's brother, little David's namesake who was himself a scholar and not a soldier like Max. Incidentally, all of Potok's maternal characters are very similar, all apparently reflections of his own mother.[9]

Again overlapping a previous novel, Potok's fifth, *The Book of Lights*, describes virtually the same period of time as *The Promise*, but its focus is also autobiographical, reflecting Potok's own years in Korea.[10] Here the key text is the Kabbalah, rather than the Talmud, although the opposition between scholars of the two texts is significant. Among this novel's issues is the theme of the "sins of the fathers," as one son deals with his own father's particular past--that Jews, attempting to end their own Holocaust, created the holocaust which the U.S. visited upon the Japanese. Potok poignantly describes Shabbat in Hiroshima, his character saying *Kaddish* for the dead (and as we now know, still dying) of Hiroshima. When this character himself dies, trying still to make peace with his father's deadly nuclear physics, the narrator once again discovers balance in the texts of tradition; texts enable him to navigate the ambiguity of post-WWII Jewish life.

Potok's third and seventh books again function together as a continuing narrative, as did his first two. *My Name is Asher Lev* and *The Gift of Asher Lev* are the most powerful and most troubling of Potok's novels, particularly for me as an outsider to Potok's world. While Potok's other novels draw me toward the Judaism he describes, since the conflicts with fundamentalism they describe find balanced resolution, the Asher Lev novels compel me to remain on the outside. In the first of these, Potok again sets up a conflict with Hasidic orthodoxy and, in this case, the *goyische* demands of art. This novel also again uses autobiography to portray Asher's overly dedicated father and long-suffering mother. The novel's central crisis is Asher's use of a crucifixion motif as the only appropriate image he can find for his mother's emotional suffering. Asher, too, is about the business of creating a balance between traditions, but in the subsequent novel, that balance is exacted at a cruel price. We again see Hasidim's continual opposition to creative art, while pictures of the theocratic Rebbe adorn classrooms, synagogue offices, homes! Asher's even more controversial painting, Potok discloses, is a portrayal of Abraham's sacrifice of Isaac, controversial because in the painting Abraham does slay his son. Just as Abraham sacrifices the life of his son, presumably to God, so Asher ultimately sacrifices his son to the Rebbe!

How much punishment must Asher undergo because he is different from the norm? In the first of these two novels the Rebbe exiles him from the Hasidic Brooklyn community and his family, and Asher moves to France. How can art as passionate as Asher's--how can reflection both intellectual and emotional--not also affect one's faith?

My own journey certainly has. Consequently, I expected more defiance from Asher against an imprisoning tradition which metaphorically eats its own children. How dare any religion or, specifically, any religious leader, vie for the life of a preschooler? And so the longing for Judaism which drew me to these seven novels now drives me into frustration and anger: Is not all this worship of Torah idolatry itself? An equivalent of the Christolatry which has perverted Christianity? How can Asher give up his son? How is *that* redemptive? Does that act of submission not rather invalidate all the defiant strength of his art? his life? Will Asher say *Kaddish* (the traditional prayer for the dead) for his son, Avrumel (Abraham!), whom he has given away?

And so my explorations have left me with but another quandary. I turned to Chaim Potok's work to attempt to find again a way into the emotions and beliefs of religious Judaism since I am no longer involved with a synagogue. Trained in theology and literature, I have found similar literary involvement an appropriate vehicle for coming to reflective knowledge and self-understanding in the past. How I admired the fathers' passion for their people, watching Max Lurie and Ariyeh Lev, for example, strive to rescue their families and friends and friends of friends from the darkness of eastern Europe, first from pogroms, then from the Holocaust. While I was deeply disturbed by the constant battling between fundamentalism and modern scholarship, I could champion Danny Saunders, Reuven Malter, and David Lurie as they made balanced commitments, claiming both their love for their religious tradition while nonetheless choosing not to avoid modern scholarship. The idea of being able to employ sound scholarship to enhance one's beloved faith is very refreshing indeed! My own efforts to work within the Judaeo-Christian tradition do not seem so different from that, as I try to balance theology and gay identity.

But by the time I had read this most recent of Potok's books, I was dismayed that the negatives seemed to outweigh the positives. At least as a whole spectrum of religious expressions, Judaism may not be any better than Christianity. The fundamentalism of Hasidic orthodoxy is deeply troubling. While the Torah, the Talmud, the Bible, or any religion's scriptures may have been divinely inspired, in the broadest possible sense of that phrase, they were certainly all humanly written, created by numerous writers and editors (redactors). They are full of contradictions. None of them was handed down from on high. Ultimately, any fundamentalism, whether Jewish, Christian, or Islamic, becomes dehumanizing. Likewise, when any religious leader gains too much control over the faithful-- whether a tzaddik or a Jim Jones--he is dangerous. Nor does any orthodoxy to my knowledge make room for gay men and lesbians. Equally problematic is the sexism inherent in any patriarchal tradition. Davita's exclusion from yeshiva honors is deeply troubling. Inwardly knowing that one is of great value is still not the same as outward recognition of one's worth.

If, then, I am again reminded that traditional Judaism has no appeal and no place for me, then, like Davita, and for that matter all Potok's leading characters, I am thrown back upon my own resources. Neither traditional Judaism nor traditional Christianity fit all my emotional or intellectual needs. I can no more choose the idolatry of Christianity (its Christology and literalized resurrection, its heteropatriarchal institutions, its ardent proselytism and thence exclusion) than I can the idolatry of Judaism (its patriarchy, its Torah worship). And yet, the hungering still persists! I again find myself between the prongs of my inherited tradition: neither Jewish nor Christian, and not really Jewish-Christian or post-Christian as others have helped me label myself and my theological work. What I am learning is that I do not like labels, that I do not need an institution, that living and thinking and believing at the margins is in fact the most appropriate place for me. And I am learning this again. Reminding myself of this again.

In my quest for community, as in my earlier quest for a lover, I have discovered community "right in my own back yard." Community is not a matter of institutional forms; it is not a matter of numbers. It does not necessarily depend upon gay/lesbian political or religious organizations, AIDS support organizations, leather clubs, recreational groups or choruses or athletic leagues. Community depends on the individuals who comprise it. I have found a community where quality is more important than quantity: a community of two, whose lives embrace our jobs, our home, our two dogs, four goldfish, a garden overflowing in tomatoes, the birds at the feeder, the flowers we have sown, the yard we mow and tend. This community is also an inclusive, nonheteropatriarchal community without gender roles, but with arms to embrace friends, supportive kinship family, and some larger gay community involvement. It is also strong enough to stand defiantly against anti-gay/lesbian discrimination, to demand recognition and rights for gay couples, to protect us from the continuing homophobia of society, church and synagogue, and even certain blood relationships. Our constructed family has become our true community, rather than our kinship families or our religious traditions of origin. This is the community we are creating and it is god/ess with us.

This special community is also a trustworthy place for (re)gaining one's perspective. As such it is my quiet sanctuary for looking again at both the Christian and the Jewish sides of my heritage. This most recent wrestling with my religious identity--and my perhaps not unexpected (re)affirmation of the goodness of not falling into any ready category--prompts me in turn to reassess my religious beliefs and those traditional ritual moments which have meaning for me. If my theology is more Christianly constructed, increasingly the ritual moments and holidays which are most meaningful to me are Jewishly constructed ones. Both of these require reexamination. And I am deeply thankful to Chaim Potok for proving the catalyst, and to his novels for proving the passageway into these activities of reappraisal.

Importantly, I am also reminded by the Asher Lev novels that I must not repeat myself. If I must paraphrase my previous work, because I still believe much of what I have already written, I must attempt to cast it in new forms. And, just as important, I must draw only upon those images and symbols which are legitimately my own. I am not Jewish and I was not raised in a Jewish home or synagogue; so, especially when I look to Jewish images, I must acknowledge my fragmentary acquaintanceship with them, limited to my brief participation in our gay/lesbian synagogue and to the handful of things which I have read. Thus are my theology and my beliefs woven of only the intellectually trustworthy fragments remaining to me from Christianity and my ritual life woven of only the fragments of Judaism which I have discovered as an empathetic outsider. For me, theologian of the margins, these fragile fragments must suffice to weave a whole cloth for my own life and spiritual needs.

(ii) Scholarship & Belief

...A reminder. ...I must not merely repeat myself, but paraphrase, recast in new forms, in the new context of searching through intellectual complexities for the simplicity of faith--a multilayered process, a distillation. So, I look to my own starting places, visiting them afresh from the vantage point of this *moment, seeking out what I really believe. And this becomes the first stage in my efforts to "keep it simple," to find among the fragments that which suffices....*

THE DIVINE

My coming out as a theological writer resulted both from my immersion in feminist studies and texts and from my involvement with a number of ardent feminists in Atlanta's gay/lesbian synagogue. More recently, as I have worked on issues of masculine socialization,[11] I have been reminded again that how we image the divine is crucial for men as well as for women. For gay men in particular, given the conditional and often rejecting relationships we experience with our own fathers, fathergod images in our religious tradition(s) have reinforced an alienation between gay men and our spirituality. At the same time, I have also come to realize the extent to which *all* our images for the divine are metaphorical; *in no case* should our images be literalized. To literalize our images of the divine, or of our experiences of the divine in our lives, is itself a form of idolatry. Whenever our tradition has literalized images of maleness, dualistic salvation, or exclusivity, the tradition has been guilty of just such idolatry!

Therefore, in opposition to all heteropatriarchal religious imagery, I want to affirm the divine as a pangendered and pansexual energy which I experience as personal and pluriform throughout my life. I want to further insist that, not only is an all-encompassing inclusivity of gender and sexuality important for understanding god/ess, but also that loving, caring, even orgasmic sexuality should be held together in our theological imagery and in our spirituality with wholeness, nurturance, independence, and creativity. Importantly, to restore sexuality to our images and concepts of god/ess is one way of also affirming people, especially those people who have been marginalized for their gender (women) or for their sexuality (gay men and lesbians).[12]

However, not only is god/ess a pangendered and pansexual energy, but the divine is also a radically horizontal energy, a presence permeating every aspect of our lives in a pluriformity of ways. Most importantly, in the midst of homophobia, anti-gay/lesbian violence, and AIDS, god/ess is a co-suffering and intimate companion who is actualized and embodied in our assumption of responsibility for ourselves and for one another--in our assumption of social responsibility and in our efforts to empower and to care for one another. God/ess and people are *interdependent*; neither can come into fullest being without the other. Such a divine companion is not only intimately bound up in human decisions and actions; s/he also suffers both human injustice and natural evil, with us in the here and now of our experience.[13] God/ess is our anger at injustice and our prophetic empowerment--in word and deed--to seek justice in our lives and to nurture the lives of our friends who struggle with AIDS.

Taken altogether as motifs from gay liberation theology-informing-faith, these concerns mean that god/ess embraces in godself the entire spectrum of gender and gender expressions, of sexuality and sexual expressions. God/ess is inherently sexual and fecund (orgasmic, creative, aesthetic) and gay men and lesbians represent valuable and divinely loved embodiments of the pluriformity of the divine nature. Neither genderless nor sexless, then, god/ess is an ultimately personal, radically horizontal, and intimately present co-suffering companion and advocate of the marginalized. Albeit with limited powers to rescue us from tragedy, god/ess nonetheless has an infinite capacity for empowering us as we assume responsibility for responding to tragedy and for creating justice. God/ess is a limited, yet prophetically empowering companion whose own eroto-creative urge is toward human responsibility and toward healthy, mutual relationships between godself and people, between people themselves, and between people and the earth. God/ess is a nurturant companion with us in oppression and tragedy who, through us, stands prophetically over-against hatred, oppression, and exploitation.[14]

My affirmations to this point are admittedly closely akin to the scholarship of process theology, especially my affirmations of divine limitations and, hence, of our experience of both divine impotence *and* divine co-suffering, even empowerment, in the silence of seeming godforsakenness. I have come to realize over the years, however, that such a view is not entirely satisfying. Although human evil, understood as failures of human responsibility, makes sense according to this view, natural evils such as the tragedy of AIDS remain problematic. Theoretical concepts of evil as resistance to the divine reinforce dualism (god/ess vs. evil) and are thus troublesome for my increasingly monotheistic point of view. But, to speak from a strictly monotheistic perspective implies that divine pluriformity must also include the possibility (the risk) of evil. And that raises other, more difficult questions: Does that make god/ess somehow *responsible* for the existence of evil, whether in nature or in human actions? Does that make the divine responsible in some manner for AIDS? How does this possibility affect the worship-worthiness of the divine?

I am left reaffirming that, ultimately, responsibility and response-ability still fall squarely upon our human shoulders. At best, we can acknowledge the limited nature of the divine and the realities of tragedies such as AIDS, and go on as best we can--befriended and empowered as we take responsibility for making a difference. We must love even a limited god/ess--or alternatively, that mysterious and pluriform Oneness which encompasses even the possibility of evil and suffering--and go on as best we can, affirming also that the One who embraces all possibilities also stands with us in our suffering and yearns with us for healing, for wholeness, for justice, and for the good.

Recently, Ron Long of Hunter College has offered an alternative for this dilemma in his two essays above. The issue of divine limitations and/or divine responsibility for evil is only an issue if we are still conceptualizing the divine as creator, as original perfect source. To do so, of course, risks falling back into traditional notions of divine omnipotence, omniscience, and omni-goodness. Long's alternative recommends relinquishing our conceptualization of god/ess as something acting in the past (as creator or first cause), and, rather, to understand god/ess as the energy of prophetic resistance (in the present) and the energy of hope (toward future liberational outcomes). This moves our imagery for the divine away from the personal toward something more abstract, something even more dependent upon human responsibility--human action to make it so. Our resistance creates and enables our hope. Long's faith in the liberational potential of the human turns traditional concepts of faith upside-down: No longer do we hope because we believe, we believe because we hope.

I believe Ron Long is correct. I believe that I am, too. At the risk of admitting that the simplicity of belief need not always perfectly coincide with the rationality of scholarship, I want to reaffirm both/and thinking, here. I want to affirm that god/ess is a creative energy, alongside us in the present instant, not in some primordial, omni-perfect past, and that, as such, god/ess is limited by the pluriformity of the Oneness which *is* godself as well as by human failures. But, even more importantly, god/ess is the embodied energy of persons prophetically resisting oppression, the embodied energy of persons working to make that which is hoped for a reality. God/ess is the embodied energy of gay/lesbian defiance before homophobia, exclusion, and anti-gay/lesbian violence. God/ess is the embodied energy of those gay men and lesbians who do not wait for someone else to correct injustice and to create justice, but who demand and create justice now, even in the midst of unjust structures. God/ess is the embodied energy of all those persons, gay or non-gay, who are responding with compassion for others during the AIDS crisis. Finally, and perhaps unlike my colleague Ron Long, above, I would insist that I experience this energy of creative resistance and hope as something *personal,* as something which depends upon my prayers and my gratitude just as much as upon my actions. I believe the divine needs me, needs us, just as much as I/we need god/ess woven into and through our lives and our actions.

And so I am led to reaffirm that the theological process of struggling to resolve the problem of evil (theodicy) is very much connected to the theological process of discerning the interrelationship of divine activity and human responsibility. God/ess is as limited by the randomness of naturally occurring evil as s/he is by human freedom and responsibility. And, yet, god/ess is not absent, either. Human action and human responsibility, human resistance and human hope, are the location or locus of divine activity. By our actions of resistance and hope, we in fact bring god/ess into being! In turn, god/ess' present creative empowerment, in addition to divine co-suffering companionship, lies in the hope for redemptive change which is embodied in responsible actions, actions which stand in prophetic judgment upon any present structures and actions which blame the victim of tragedy or injustice.[15]

Importantly, these efforts to reconceptualize god/ess and to penetrate theodicy work against any idolatrous capturing of the divine within limited images by continually forcing me to reexamine human ways of being and acting in the world. As I have said elsewhere, the focus for gay liberation theology, and thus for a liberational faith built upon that foundation, progressively becomes less about god/ess and shifts instead to that of human responsibility.[16]

THE HUMAN

The radical horizontality of god/ess and the interdependence of the divine with humanity means that *we* bear the responsibility for actualizing justice in the world. *We* bring god/ess into being, sustaining and being sustained by the divine, through our actions of right-relationship making. Thus do we discover that god/ess with us is not only a companion, but also a prophetic critic of *any* status quo which oppresses, exploits, or excludes. Because of our interdependence, we are expected to confront the realities of evil and injustice without escapism and apart from waiting for divine rescue. Taking responsible and responsive action, instead, actually brings god/ess into being, empowering us by our empowering of godself. Our encounter with the divine presence is fulfilled *only* by and in human action(s). Moreover, our capacities to respond and to act, or our failures to do so, also affect or limit divine power. We create, enable, and empower god/ess with us whenever we act responsibly, and we curtail or undermine god/ess with us whenever we fail to act or whenever we choose oppressive, exploitative, exclusive, life-denying, or otherwise "evil" actions.[17]

As a further result of radical horizontality and interdependence, our complicity in or our passivity before anti-gay/lesbian violence and homophobic oppression may actually be sinful,[18] as is any willingness on our part to accept a heterosexist, bracketed, genitally reduced sexuality as the delimiting factor of our gay/lesbian being. Gay men and lesbians are far more than just our sexuality and our sexuality itself is an erotic wholeness which encompasses far more than mere genital function. In fact, as I have argued in more than one other context,[19] we must never consider our sexuality as merely some dualistic genital function. Such genital reductionism undermines our capacity for realizing that the erotic actually *permeates* our existence, heals our lives, nurtures and sacramentalizes our relationships, and creates wholeness for us. The erotic, experienced most fully in our sexuality, demands justice or right-relationship in our most intimate partnerships, and through those right-relationships, urges us toward justice in all relationships.

Obviously, then, responsibility in the area of sexuality includes more than just safe-sex in the age of AIDS. It also means seeking the wholeness of self and of partner(s) within sexual relationships. For me, this entails a *pragmatic* choice of monogamy as the best way for my partner and I to focus, share, and nurture our intimacy and our energies-in-relationship--as we build our relationship, our home, and our lives together--also interdependent. Herein do we find wholeness and the energies, jointly shared, for our own pursuits of justice in the world. No, monogamy is not some moral absolute carved in stone and handed down from on high. It is a pragmatic value, a choice made because I believe that our sexuality, and our gay/lesbian sexuality, is sacramental and that whenever we act out sexually in non-sacramental ways and/or in ways which dehumanize our partners, then we trivialize our sexuality. Responsibility means refusing to treat ourselves or our partners as genital machines.[20]

To affirm the sacramental quality of our sexuality is part and parcel of my also reaffirming that our embodied experience is our only locus for knowing and experiencing all things, including god/ess. We know through our bodily experience--our senses, our sensuality, our eros--as well as through our embodied interactions with others.[21] As Ron Long said above, "We are our bodies." And, as a result, our knowledge of all things--of nature, of people, of god/ess--is fundamentally erotic or sensual. However, as I watch friends' embodiments diminishing under the duress of AIDS, and as I have watched my grandmother's embodiment diminishing with age, I have discovered that radically affirming ourselves as our bodies also presents difficult questions.

If we affirm our embodiedness as the only locus of our experience, including our experience and knowledge of the divine, does the diminishing of our bodily capacities also imply a corresponding diminishing decline in our spiritual capacities? Does my friend who is hearing-impaired also have an impaired knowledge of god/ess? Do impairments of whatever kind qualitatively impair the meaning of bodily-spiritual experience? Does my sick friend's spiritual awareness decline as his body weakens? Does his no longer desiring or his inability to engage in sexuality impair his bodily-spiritual experience? Is my grandmother less spiritual because she is becoming less mobile? Obviously, I do not think so.

Since our experience of our senses and our experience as bodies certainly varies, our knowledge of the world and of god/ess must also be varied. *But,* differences in our ways of experiencing god/ess and the world need not imply hierarchically *qualitative* differences. And yet, radically body-oriented theologies may risk that implication. To the contrary, it could be argued that, in a world where physical and sensory differences were not considered impairments to full participation in human existence, in a world that was fully accessible to all persons regardless of their physical/sensory condition, the pluriformity of embodied experiencing might reflect god/ess' own pluriformity. As it is, those who are physically or sensory challenged stand in prophetic judgment over against those who would exclude them or disvalue them, as well as over against those who in any way compound the suffering of those who are different. At the same time, these same impairments again confront us with the dilemma of the existence of natural evil and, as such, remind us that theodicy remains incompletely resolved.

How then do we affirm that we are our bodies while simultaneously insisting that bodily impairments do not hinder our spiritual experience? Can we affirm the positive value of a pluriformity of embodied experiencing? How do we further resolve theodicy beyond those tentatively suggested ways outlined above by myself and by Ron Long, in ways which comfort the impaired? These surely remain open questions for all persons engaged in radically this-worldly liberation theologies--loose ends requiring further exploration and reflection, reminders of the always fragmentary and incomplete nature of theology-as-activity. One thing I will affirm: Whatever our embodied and sensory condition, god/ess is with us, both in our embodiments and in our human interrelationships, here and now. Likewise, it is up to *us* to create justice and to embody compassion to all persons in all conditions of embodied life. *That* is god/ess with us.

Another, very different problem also arises in regard to radical body-affirmation. The radical assertion that "we are our bodies" may also imply that "we are nothing more than our embodied experience." Such reductionism would perforce deny any and all possibilities for any life or experience as persons beyond the limits of this life. Importantly, liberation theologies of all sorts, including gay liberation theology, need to stand firm over against eschatological theologies whose valuing of the *next* life leads to a devaluation of and disregard for this life. Such other-worldly theologies have long been used to maintain the status quo and to exploit both minority peoples and the earth itself. Theology which is radically horizontal and here and now, fusing theory with the praxis of liberation, revalues this life, this world, and this earth. Such a theological emphasis demands liberation for all peoples here and now; such a theological emphasis demands respect and healing for the earth here and now. But, at the same time, are we willing to rule out all possibilities for life after death?

Numerous alternatives abound: While apologetic writers retain a very traditional Christian hope for life after death, especially in view of the way in which AIDS has foreshortened so many lives,[22] other writers, such as Raymond Moody, have examined "near-death" experiences and their commonalities, suggesting that some clinical evidence may exist to substantiate belief in personal experience, apart from our bodies, after death.[23] Not unrelated to Moody's work is the popular belief in reincarnation--that after our experience of dying (as described by near-death patients), we exist outside embodiment until our individual energies are again embodied in another human, this-worldly existence. Of course, where and how the energies of our individual selves exist between embodiments remains an open question.

Granted, in the waning years of the 20th century, and in the face of the still monumental tasks facing all liberation theologies, any such eschatological, otherworldly hopes may appear trite if not even counterproductive. And yet, because we cannot know for certain, even a radically horizontal and body affirming theology may leave open the *possibility* for some personal experience after the demise of our current bodies, albeit without any misdirected focus on such open-endedness. One thing I will affirm: *This* life, *this* embodiment, and our embodied sensuous experience of *this* world in *this* life-time are the only reality we actually know with any certainty. It is within this life and this world that we experience god/ess with us as the divine demand and empowerment for justice for all peoples and for the earth *here and now.* Our current bodies are the loci of our experiencing, of our knowing, and of our assuming responsibility. Theoretical eschatological possibilities aside, here and now is where we meet and enable god/ess with us.

ONE OTHER THING

And then there is the figure of Jesus with which to contend. Traditional Jews will not even utter his name, let alone discuss him. Traditional Christians never cease uttering his name: His name adorns license plates, bumper

stickers, and roadside signs. His name is exploited by in-
fighting televangelists to extort millions from their loyal
viewers. We are inundated with his name. We can no
more refuse to deal with Jesus in such Christolatrous times
than we can fail to wrestle with the problem of evil in the
age of AIDS. He has been misunderstood and ignored by
his own native Judaism, while he has been idolatrously di-
vinized by post-Pauline Christians who equally misunder-
stand and distort his historical life. Such a minor figure in
the overall history of humankind and yet one whose name
and divinization have nonetheless shaped a history wrought
with antisemitism, inquisitorial witch hunts, the imperialis-
tic exploitation and genocide of non-Christian native
peoples in the Americas and elsewhere, and continuing sexism and homophobia in our own day--such a man must be
dealt with.

    Jesus was not god/ess. Jesus was not a dying-rising
god. Jesus *was* Jewish, a man who intended no break with
Judaism, a man who did not himself claim to be the messiah, although Judaism had been rife with messianic pretenders until liberal Judaism moved away from messianic
expectations in the last century.[24] Rather than breaking
with Judaism, Jesus radicalized the prophetic tradition
within Judaism, especially the norm of justice as taught by
his near contemporary Hillel, seasoning that with the Jewish apocalypticism he found among the Essenes. His death,
when it came, was a political expedient on the part of the
powerholders of his region--both Roman *and* Jewish
leaders--and was *not* the product of any ethnic group, Jewish or otherwise. There was no "Christ-killing" and therefore no legitimate Christolatrous rational for antisemitism
over the ensuing two millennia.[25]

    As for Jesus' sexuality or its meaning for gay liber-
ation theology and belief, there is no textual evidence for
celibacy or for sexual activity on his part. What we do
find, instead, is a picture of someone who was not obsessed

with sexuality, but who was able to relate to both men and women as friends first, not as sexual objects, and who was therefore able to express his love to both men and women with physical affection.[26] He was a fully human individual and a full participant in bodily, and hence sexual, human existence. He was an eclectic thinker, pulling together Hillel and the Essenes. He was a radical believer in the present demand of justice. He was an embodiment of assumed human responsibility, of resistance and hope. And that alone is enough. We do not need him to be a god or a messiah or even particularly unique.

Faith informed by liberation theology does not require such trinitarian language. As I have said elsewhere, a radically monotheistic and horizontally present divine can be self-conscious, self-reflective, and self-integrated without being split or divided against godself. The analogy of human self-relatedness and the experience of god/ess' horizontally intimate relation in history are sufficient.[27] That god/ess permeates the cosmos and is embodied in every life and in every just relationship is sufficient. Indeed, especially as regards Jesus, we are again reminded that all theological language is metaphorical and should not be idolatrously literalized. Our language is metaphorical and is not meant to imply real, verifiable historical events. We should not literalize the metaphor of resurrection; the crucifixion alone may well be the better symbolic locus of god/ess' co-suffering empowerment in the silence of godforsakenness.[28] We should not literalize the metaphor of incarnation; we are all embodiments of the divine energy, insofar as we assume responsibility for justice-seeking and -making in our lives and our relationships. A messiah is not required to make resistance, justice-seeking action, and responsibility realities in the present. Our own lives are sufficient, if we will but assume responsibility for embodying god/ess, to one another and to the world.

...Even while we elaborate our faith in systematic details, that which we seek to hold in our intellectual hands disappears from sight. The details will not hold the divine. We may never resolve the problem of evil so that our solution encompasses every dilemma. We may need more time to consider the implications of radically affirming our embodiment. And yet, I know the demand of justice for all oppressed persons and our exploited planet is imperative. I also know that even though god/ess depends upon us to make godself manifest in the world, god/ess is not just a creation of human minds. Even an interdependent, radically horizontal, here and now god/ess has reality for me. Just as the energy of a relationship requires tending as some reality over and above the two participants in a commitment, so, too, is god/ess that energy over and above the sum of the parts, a Oneness knitting it all together, permeating all things, waiting on and empowering our commitments to justice and right-relation. We bring god/ess into being even as the divine sustains our lives. And that, simply, is indeed sufficient.

(iii) Holidays, Rituals, & Prayers

Although I obviously consider myself a *religious* person, I am not *ritually* oriented. When I previously indicated that certain rituals might be of religious significance for the gay/lesbian community, for example, I reflected upon those already existing subcultural rituals and holidays which might disclose spiritual significance for us, as well as upon already established religious occasions which we might appropriate for their latent gay/lesbian meaningfulness.[29] Now that I am again led to consider the related issues of prayer, rituals, and religious holidays, I am reminded of the extent to which my own life has progressively disposed of all these, except private, informal prayer. Indeed, I practice my own idiosyncratic piety, not in the Wesleyan sense of my upbringing and seminary training, but rather somewhat in the sense Ron Long described above--an honoring which is compatible with the acknowledgement of fault or limitation in the revered object, albeit an honoring which for me is also worship. Consequently, my ruminations over my connections to Judaism, rather than my Christian upbringing and training, constitute the impetus which has now brought me back to these issues.

Moving away from trinitarian beliefs almost inevitably led me to abandon all Christian holidays and rituals. One simply cannot avoid the Christocentrism in the vast majority of them. Christmas provides one glaring example. Obviously, without the Christolatrous divinization of Jesus, such a holiday would be meaningless. Moreover, Christmas has been theologically orchestrated from the beginning. The gospels of Matthew and Luke present two distinct Christmas narratives which the popular tradition has naively fused into one; neither of these is historically reliable, insofar as both of them are theological constructions consistent with the particular writer's larger purposes. (For a clearer example of a theologically constructed narrative of Jesus'/Christ's origins, one only need examine the opening of the gospel of John.) Moreover, the birth of Jesus, originally celebrated in March, was moved by an early church council to December 25th--heretofore the liturgical calendar had his birth and death uncomfortably too close together! And the western, competitive and commercial abomination which this holiday has become requires little elaboration, although it certainly should evoke our contempt. Also noteworthy is the fact that Jesus' birthday celebration now coincides, roughly, with Chanukah, Kwanzaa, and, in the northern hemisphere, with every other winter solstice holiday. Perhaps beneath the various layers of mythic euphemism and western commercialization, the only significant holiday at this time of year really is the solstice--the death and rebirth of the sun, the change of seasons, and the hope for a distant but dependable spring three months hence.

Easter may be even more difficult for the monotheist. I have written elsewhere of the difficulties of literalizing resurrection. Just as no trustworthy historical evidence exists to pinpoint Jesus' birthday (and certainly not in December), no historically reliable data exists to support a literal resurrection. "Resurrection" is a metaphor for his followers' experience of his still living influence for them. The far more important day to remember in this "passion narrative" may rather be Good Friday, including Jesus' abandonment by his disciples, his crucifixion, and, therein, his experience of both divine abandonment and divine co-suffering and empowerment.[30] Again, an overlap with Judaism occurs, since Jesus' "last supper" is most likely a Passover Seder meal. Not surprisingly, both holidays occur as nearly in conjunction with the spring equinox as do Christmas/Chanukah occur in conjunction with the winter solstice. The real holiday beneath the mythic layers is thus revealed--the welcoming of spring, the cyclic renewal of the earth and, hence, of the human psyche and our will to live.

Having thus demythologized the two major holidays of Christianity, we may still find that other potentially meaningful holidays remain within the Jewish side of our two pronged Judaeo-Christian tradition. Granted, when I study my Hebrew year calendar, I realize I recognize few of the names. Some of those with which I am familiar are problematic; others are not. Those holidays which are most cyclical are also the ones with which my own experience best resonates. Holiest of all holidays is the Sabbath-- Shabbat; when Shabbat falls during any other holiday period, it is always most revered. For me, Shabbat represents an important separation from the world of work; it signals the beginning of the weekend and, for that reason alone, is cause to give thanks to god/ess. It is a time for my spouse and I to have a meal away from home, to sleep a little later, to spend time with our yard and dogs and each other, without the constraints of our scheduled weeks. Shabbat for us is actually a two-day reprieve, refreshingly occuring every week. A different cycle is represented by Rosh Chodesh, the monthly cycle of the new moon and of Hebrew months. Again, the resonance is with the cyclical nature of our lives. It is also a time for recognizing both our feminine aspects as gay men and the value of women-only space (physically *and* spiritually) for our lesbian sisters.

From the cycles of the week and the month, the Hebrew calendar yields itself to the cycle of the year. Again, I would suggest a cosmic holiday beneath the religious value of Rosh Hashana--the fall equinox, the harvest. Moreover, as an academic who has lived by the school year since kindergarten, I find that it really does coincide with a new year. And our culture is replete with similar new year imagery, from new car style unveilings to new television and fine arts seasons. Not just academics begin new years in the fall! In conjunction with Rosh Hashana, however, is one of the most problematic of holidays in the Jewish calendar--Yom Kippur/Kol Nidre. While the solemnness of the Day of Atonement includes the important activities of forgiving and reconciling--that divine forgiveness depends upon our righting the wrongs we have commited and forgiving those who have wronged us--and while the Yizkor memorial service importantly lifts up the memories of those who have died--a very significant activity especially under the spectre of AIDS in our community, the underlying theme of divine predestination is hard to accept. The image of a divine "book of life" wherein the names of those who will die in the coming year are inscribed suggests, again in view of AIDS, that god/ess determines the deaths of our loved ones in advance. Such choosing can only seem cruel! Better that our new year begin only with reconciling and remembering, as well as with a renewed commitment on all our parts to keep alive those whom we have lost to AIDS in our own future-ward living.

Apart from these clearly cyclical holidays, other days within the Jewish calendar are somewhat less important. While Chanukah (despite its minor holiday status [it clearly is not a Jewish "equivalent" of Christmas] and its original context in a military victory) does provide us with a moment to join in solidarity with all persons celebrating light in the midst of winter's oncoming darkness, Simchat Torah seems as idolatrous as Easter. Worshipping the Torah as something divinely revealed is something which I simply cannot do. And, as an outsider, I cannot consent to the theme of chosenness. I will keep Chanukah, I will light candles to brighten the winter, but I will set aside Torah celebrations with those Christian holidays I can no longer honor.

No doubt the two holidays in either prong of our tradition which are most meaningful to me are Pesach (Passover) and Yom HaShoah (Holocaust Remembrance). As a celebration of liberation, Passover cannot help but be symbolically important for gay men and lesbians. Pesach clearly symbolizes and remembers divine historical empowerment of one particular marginalized people to assume human responsibility and to enact human liberation. Its tremendous power as a symbol, however, transcends its particularity and points to god/ess as liberator--to the divine urge for justice--on behalf of *any* marginalized group. Pesach celebrates not only god/ess' liberating power in history, but god/ess' liberating co-empowerment on behalf of all people still on the margins. It also symbolically signifies god/ess as the grounding and source of empowerment for any people to actively seek their own liberation. God/ess is not just with the powerless, but is actually one of them/us. God/ess sanctifies the defiance of all those who suffer human injustice (homophobia) or nature's unfairness (AIDS) or pre-mature suffering and death (AIDS, anti-gay/

lesbian violence). That blessing of defiance, or resistance in Ron Long's words, creates hope and demands that we take responsibility for not just enduring, but for persevering both in our compassion for those struggling with AIDS and in our quest for justice and for liberation for all people.[31]

As Pesach is a celebration of our defiant urge toward liberation, so Yom HaShoah is a remembrance of those who have fallen along the way, especially of those who died under the Nazis. As a plethora of research has shown, not only did six million Jews die during the Third Reich, but so did some quarter million gay men. Among the few formal prayers I find meaningful is one which honors these lives and therefore deserves reprinting in this context:

> ...We are called upon to remember not only the six million, but another quarter million, those gay people, primarily gay men, who vanished in the Holocaust because of how and whom they loved. Their sacrifice to the demons of power, war, and sexism we must redeem by remembering. While we remember their pain, we would also transform that pain, through remembering, into the energies of liberation.

> *In the presence of eyes which witnessed the slaughter,*
> *which saw the oppression the heart could not bear,*
> *and as witness the heart that once taught compassion,*
> *until the days came to pass that crushed human feeling,*
> *I have taken an oath:*
> *To remember it all, to remember, not once to forget!*
> *An oath: Not in vain the terror and the fear.*
> *An oath: Not in vain our lovers vanished, gay people slain.*
> *An oath: Lest from this we learned nothing!*
> *Our music and laughter, our revelry, camp, and dance were*
>   *exchanged*
> *for the sounds of the trains, the smoke of the chimneys.*
> *Our beauty, our youth, our vigor slowly worked to death;*

*our sexuality mocked, both suddenly and gradually taken from
    us;*
our gayness wisked away like smoke and ash.
Because invisible, the nations could not or would not save us.
Because remaining outcast, restitution was denied us.

As we watched our lovers taken from us, as our hearts and
souls were exhausted, we questioned you, god/ess: Are you
impotent? Absent? Do you hate us, too?

*Answer us, god/ess, answer us as we remember our affliction;
be mindful of our plea, and hear our supplication.*

Yet in the dark and smoke-filled silence, in the weariness at
the verge of death, we found you weeping among us; we realized your delight in variety, in both gay and non-gay; we realized that you had created us, your gay and lesbian children.

*You, O god/ess, answer us in time of trouble; your love is our
comfort; you rescue and redeem in time of distress.*

The dynamics of the holocaust had to attack gay people, and
homosexuality in general, which questions the opposition of
the sexes and threatens male supremacy. Even the dreadful
suffering that gay people have experienced has its good side, *if*
we learn to read it correctly. To be attacked by an enemy such
as Nazism shows that there must indeed be something important and progressive in our particular sexuality.

*We give thanks to you, O god/ess, for claiming and loving us
as your children, to embody your presence in suffering, in silence, and in action. We rejoice in your gifts of who we are
and in the tasks of liberation which you have given to us. You
are indeed the redeemer of all the oppressed. Blessed is the
eternal one, the source of freedom, the empowerment for liberation.*[32]

So logically, then, does formal prayer emerge from religious holiday rituals, even for me, even from those few rituals which remain meaningful for me. The one other holiday whose prayers hold some lasting value for me, as a theologian on the margins apart from *any* institutions, is Shabbat and, specifically, the Friday evening Shabbat service which does *not* include a Torah reading. While these reflections are *not* intended as a prayerbook, certain prayers or combinations of prayers from an early gay/lesbian prayerbook remain important for me, insofar as they reflect my own theological and spiritual values.[33] I believe they may also resonate with the experience of other gay men and lesbians as well and are therefore important to record in this context. One of the caveats in that prayerbook also remains instructive for my renderings of these few prayers as well: Because god/ess is beyond form and gender--or because god/ess is pangendered and pansexual, beyond the duality of the male/female opposition--the language of prayer should reflect this with gender-neutral, inclusive language. My renderings of these prayers, therefore, not only attempt to reflect my own theology and spirituality (beliefs), but also attempt to employ this caveat in an even more thoroughgoing fashion than did the prayerbook itself, eschewing not only gender-laden pronouns, but also hierarchical terms, dualistic concepts, and chosenness motifs wherever possible.[34]

Traditionally, the Shabbat evening ritual begins with welcoming in this special holiday. An appropriate prayer might include:

> The Sabbath is not a day for the soul alone; it is meant for the body as well. Holiness does not mean removal from the world, but the sanctification of it. We come before you, O god/ess, your gay sons and lesbian daughters. We come to add our voices to those of others in worship and in prayer. (Kabbalat Shabbat I, III)

or:

> On the Sabbath, we are reminded that justice is our duty and a
> better world our goal. Therefore, we welcome Shabbat: Day
> of rest; day of wonder; day of peace. (Kabbalat Shabbat VIII)

Shabbat officially begins with the lighting of candles, again
the evoking of light as darkness falls, not unlike the symbolic evocation of light in winter at Chanukah:

> Blessed is god/ess, energy of the cosmos, who hallows us with
> mitzvot (the demands of justice), and joins us as we kindle the
> lights of Shabbat.

Later in a Shabbat service comes what is considered the
central prayer of Judaism, the *Shema*. Importantly, this
prayer makes no request of god/ess; it only affirms that
god/ess is one. Among the preludes to the *Shema* is one
which speaks specifically to gay men and lesbians:

> As gay men and lesbians, we often feel compelled to pretend
> to be that which we are not, to present ourselves in ways
> which are not truthful, and sometimes, with outright lies.

> *But as we stand before you, our words and our thoughts speed
> to one who knows them before we utter them. We do not have
> to tell untruths to you as we often feel forced to do in the
> straight world. We know we cannot lie in your presence.*

> May our worship help us to practice truth in speech and in
> thought before you, to ourselves, and before one another; and
> may we finally complete our liberation so that we no longer
> feel the need to practice evasions and deceits.

> *God/ess, purify our hearts to serve you in truth.* (Shema V)

The best known portion of the main body of the *Shema* it-self is meaningful, not literally of course, but rather in its symbolizing the centrality of the divine energy throughout the cosmos and in our own lives--an affirmation important enough to me to have hung on the doorpost of our home:

> You shall love god/ess with all your heart, with all your soul, and with all your might. And these words which I command you this day shall be upon your heart. You shall teach them diligently to your children, and shall speak of them when you sit in your house, and when you walk on the road, when you lie down, and when you rise up. You shall bind them for a sign upon your hand, and they shall be for frontlets between your eyes. You shall write them upon the doorposts of your house and upon your gates.

After the *Shema* is said, every service recalls the liberation from Egypt. And thus, importantly, does liberation run throughout all gatherings of Jewish prayer. In and of itself, this constant reminder of god/ess' power as liberating energy alongside us evokes the same empowerment as Pesach. As gay men and lesbians we are never without a companion in our struggle for our fullest liberation.

At a later point in traditionally constructed services, comes a time for personal meditation. Numerous suggested prayers and a concluding prayer are offered to worshippers. As I have dealt with the loss of friends to AIDS, the changes in previous relationships (and the ill feelings which those too often create), and the other elements in my life, the most meaningful of these to me is the following:

> O god/ess, keep my tongue from evil and my lips from speaking guile. Be my support when grief silences my voice, and my comfort when woe bends my spirit. Implant humility in my soul, and strengthen my heart with perfect faith in you. Help me to be strong in temptation and trial and to be patient

and forgiving when others wrong me. Guide me by the light of your counsel, that I may ever find strength in you.

May the words of our mouths and the meditations of our hearts be acceptable to you, O god/ess, our rock and our redeemer. May god/ess who establishes peace, grant peace to us and to all the world. Amen. (Personal Amida III, IV)

At this point in a service, a sermon might traditionally be given, or in more informal settings, a discussion engaged in by everyone. After which, as a service draws to a close, come other opportunities for prayers. Several of these resonate with my experience as a gay person and also reaffirm my commitments to gender parity and to feminist ideals:

Let us give praise to god/ess and adore the energy of the cosmos.

As gay men and lesbians, we sometimes feel compelled to hide the qualities that distinguish us from others: our love for each other, our heritage of creativity spanning the milenia, our unique attributes with which we, in your image, were created.

But this cannot affect our inner resolve to honor and fulfill our special purpose, to live out this wonderful and unknowable design, in which each of us has a part to play.

Let us, therefore, express our deep gratitude to the god/ess of Abraham and Sarah, of Moses and Miriam, of David and Jonathan, of Ruth and Naomi, the holy one, of blessed name. (Aleynu I, II)

May the time not be distant, god/ess, when all peoples abandon bigotry and cease the blasphemy of calling on your name to justify oppression and hatred. On that day, as we recognize that we are all brothers and sisters, your realm shall be established on earth and the word of your prophet shall be fulfilled: "The Eternal will abide with us forever and ever." (Aleynu III)

Among all the various prayers within the evening service and those included in the eclectic prayerbook which I find meaningful, are two prayers which surpass all the others in their significance for me as a gay person. One of those is a "prayer for the end of hiding," used after the group discussion. Its value is self-evident:

> As gay men and lesbians, we are aware of the loss of integrity we suffer due to pressures from the larger society. We often feel compelled into a dishonest presentation of ourselves, to ourselves and to others. The gay men and lesbians who feel they must pretend to be something that they are not, the Jews who feel they must be alienated from their tradition and community to win larger acceptance, both are victims of a theft of identity and integrity committed by the sexual or religious majority.

> Loving god/ess, we ask that our hiding draw to an end, that we no longer feel we have to pretend, to promise falsely, to renounce ourselves, and that our fullest creative expression as Jews and as gay people be among the blessings you bestow upon us. Amen.

The other of these especially significant prayers is the *Mourner's Kaddish.* While this prayer contains no reference to death as such, it instead affirms the significance of life, it sanctifies our lives as one with god/ess, and it recommits our lives, on behalf of those who have died, to our duties to compassion and justice. Among the preludes to the *Kaddish* proper, are words which remember those gay men and lesbians for whom there is no one to recite this prayer, thus including and remembering *all* our brothers and sisters:

Our thoughts turn now to those who have died, our own loved ones, those dear to our friends and neighbors, the martyrs of our people whose graves are unmarked, those lesbians and gay men for whom there is no one to recite *Kaddish*, and those of every race and nation whose lives have been a blessing to humanity, enriching our own lives. God/ess, remember today our gay and lesbian brothers and sisters who were martyred in years past, those who were murdered by fanatics in the Middle Ages, those who perished in the Holocaust, those struck down in our own city and our own time, those driven to despair at living in a world that hated them because of their love for one another and who took their own lives, and those who have wasted their lives by suppressing their true natures and by refraining from sharing their love with one another. O god/ess, accept the holy sacrifice of these martyrs, and help us bring an end to hate and oppression of every kind. (Mourners Kaddish I, II, III)

The *Kaddish* itself follows, the prayer of praise and remembrance which is important to me for all those whom my spouse and I have lost to AIDS, and which is also important to me that I should say it for my spouse or he should say it for me, when our time also comes:

Magnified and sanctified be god/ess' great name. May the dominion of god/ess [a just world] be established during your life and during your days, speedily and at a near time, and let us say: Amen.

Let god/ess' great name be blessed forever and to all eternity.

Blessed and praised and glorified and exalted and extolled and honored and adored and lauded be the name of the holy one, though god/ess be above all the blessings and hymns, praises and songs, which are uttered in the world, and let us say: Amen.

May there be abundant peace and a good life for us and for all,
and let us say: Amen.

May god/ess who makes peace make peace for us and for all
the world, and let us say: Amen.

These, then, are the prayers which I have borrowed from
Judaism--from gay and lesbian Judaism--because they resonate within my own life, within my own humble efforts
not only to do theology, but to create for myself a credo, a
way of being in the world as a faithful, faith-filled individual. My translations into gender-free language may differ
from the words the tradition or others might choose; that I
would pray these prayers at all, even in the privacy of my
own heart, may offend traditional believers, but that does
not undercut their value for my own spirituality. More importantly, I do not believe that "prepared" prayers can ever
substitute for our own reflections shared with the cosmos--
with god/ess. My morning prayers, for example, shared
toward the growing day as I go to work, always include a
thanksgiving for the new day and its opportunities, a
thanksgiving for my spouse and our home together, pleas
on behalf of whatever crisis or crises have appeared in recent news, pleas on behalf of all those dealing with HIV
and AIDS, whether as patients, as survivors, or in grief, and
finally a shared hope that I can be a contributing energy to
god/ess' own energy during the day. This is how I begin
my day.

Increasingly, then, the theologian's task is neither to
prescribe or proscribe, but is rather simply to share one's
own pilgrimage, one's own personal growth. That is, of
course, an ongoing process. To bring this part of that process to a close, I can best offer what has always been my
favorite benediction, the one we used to close every choir
concert in college, as well as the one frequently used by
gay and lesbian synagogues:

May god/ess bless you and keep you.
May god/ess show you kindness and be gracious unto you.
May god/ess bestow favor upon you and grant you peace.
Amen.

(iv) Epilogue & Credo

As I have worked through the intellectual intricacies of my own scholarship--the academic study of religion and of theology--and as I have examined rituals, holidays, and prayers, I know that I may *appear* to have little left by which to construct a workable "lavender credo." My deconstructions and reconstructions are certainly most heterodox, even defiantly asserting my disdain for institutions, my distrust of virtually every inherited, traditional form and creed. All too often, such details--givens proffered with putative authority--utterly dismay me and, at times, even disgust me when they appear to constrain and dehumanize rather than to liberate human beings. Family, friends, readers, too, perhaps, worry over the "salvation of my soul" as if it were but some dualistic disembodiment.

And yet, for all my heresy--so called by the traditions whose details I must either dismiss, deconstruct or eclectically rearrange--I know that I am nonetheless a deeply devout believer. Forego labeling my beliefs. I have a credo nonetheless. "I believe" and I do so passionately. All theology risks becoming but an academic exercise in face of the pluriform Oneness whom I affirm, love, worship--that cosmic Mystery always just out of reach of our metaphors. Theologies can become so complicated when, instead, bottom-line *liberational* faith can really be a very simple matter--how I experience god/ess in the everydayness of life.

With that in mind, I name as god/ess the all-permeating, pluriform energy *which I experience as personal*, as far more nurturing, maternal, companion-like, than as any-

thing masculine or judgmental. For those who pay attention, history and our actions in history, however mundane,
carry their own inherent judgment, self-criticism, and cor-
rectives--to which we should pay heed. For those times
when we do not hear, then, yes, god/ess is also a prophetic,
curmudgeonly energy, strongly yet lovingly reproving, the
energy of idealism and of justice-seeking action, the energy
of defiant righteous anger in the pursuit of wholeness-
making justice. Yet, it is as companion that I most often
find god/ess energy in my life--the muse-like energies I invoke to join my writing, the Socratic energies I invite into
every classroom, the Hippocratic energies I pray abide with
friends who struggle with AIDS. I also name as god/ess
the object of my gratitude for every new morning, for my
spouse and our relationship, for our home and our constructed family. God/ess is the quiet of morning, new days,
new beginnings. God/ess is the energy of love-making and
coupled playfulness. God/ess is the caring and healing energy embodied in people acting compassionately before
tragedy--before AIDS--and in my spouse's ability to give
himself so easily to others and to the needs of others. Yes,
god/ess may be limited, unable to rescue; but, more importantly, god/ess is able to share pain, grief, recovery, joy.
God/ess is the energy of my own tenacity.

Ultimately, my credo is not something terribly so-
phisticated. It's just "how it is with me," an invitation to
share, to talk, to enjoy together the simplicity of pluriform
Oneness.[35] And, after all, what other details do we really
need? Certainly not the confusing, confining, defining, oft-
dehumanizing details of orthodoxies and their institutional
(dis)embodiments. The details of our own lives are more
than enough to suffice, to testify, to embody god/ess with
us. Over a decade ago, Sheila Collins poignantly described
just this presentness, this intimate horizontality of the divine in our lives, as the point from which we begin doing

theology, from which we begin to find our voice for saying what we believe:

> Theology begins with our stories: What we do with our time; how we feel about our families, our friends, our coworkers, our bosses; how we feel about money and who gets it; what we do when we get up in the morning; how we make it through the day; what pains us, enrages, us, saddens and humiliates us; what makes us laugh; what enlightens and empowers us; what keeps us holding on in moments of despair; where we find separation and alienation; where we find true community and trust.[36]

Yes, our lives--our own pluriform, fragmented, weavings toward wholeness, disclose the simplicity, the mystery beyond words and metaphors ... Listen! See! God/ess with us!

God/ess with us in the still-waking-up half-light of a new day, the red-orange orb of the sun just at the horizon's edge and in the dappled sunlight an hour later, filtered through the trees and over the green, green lawns and leaves. God/ess with us through the varied light of the day, the sunbathing caress of noon, the twilight reflected back in the dome of an urban sky, or the deep star-lit blue of my native mountains. God/ess with us embodied in the neighbor-lady who stays with my aging and now ailing grandmother, helping her to walk and to exercise, preparing her meals, being her companion. God/ess with us embodied in every gay man, lover, lesbian-friend who provides the basics of committed companionship for a loved one living and dying with AIDS. God/ess with us embodied in the love of my spouse for me, of me for him, in the humor and playfulness of high emotions, in the patient waiting-through of low, often silent emotions, in our work together on the yard and garden, flowers and vegetables, in our dogs and their affectionate neediness, in a special friend sharing the intimacy of a meal at our table, and in the privacy of our love-making, sometimes surprisingly quick, sometimes lazily slow--god/ess with us in ecstasy, in blessing, in loving and simply in being there. God/ess with us in caring for and about friends who are ill or dying ... or, now, remembered ... and god/ess with us, given voice by a gay men's chorus singing our defiance, our love for one another, our perseverance. God/ess with us in gay pride, in mass commitment ceremonies, in protests, sit-ins, die-ins for our rights as a people, as persons--god/ess with us, permeating every aspect of our lives.

Both source and resistance and hope. Alpha and omega, as the metaphor says. Gentle mother, reproving friend, truest companion, embodied in and by our lives to stand alongside us. God/ess with us. Come. Affirm yourself. Love your community. Embrace the Oneness. Celebrate the heresy. God/ess with us! Amen!

---

[1]J. Michael Clark, *A place to start: Toward an unapologetic gay liberation theology* (Dallas: Monument Press, 1989).

[2]Nell Morton, *The journey is home* (Boston: Beacon Press, 1985), p. xxv.

[3]For the best example of what will remain for some time the most compassionate, albeit still futile, of denominational studies on human sexuality, including gay/lesbian sexuality, see: Special Committee on Human Sexuality (John J. Carey, Chair), *Keeping body and soul together: Sexuality, spirituality, and social justice.* Report to the 203rd General Assembly, Presbyterian Church (USA), Baltimore, 4-12 June 1991, 196 pp. The commissioners to the General Assembly did not adopt this "majority report" *nor* did it adopt a conservative "minority report." The General Assembly instead adopted a "pastoral letter" (dated 11 June 1991) reaffirming the denomination's commitment to the authority of scripture and to the sanctity of the heterosexual marriage covenant. The letter also carefully stated, "We continue to abide by the 1978 and 1979 positions of the Presbyterian Church on

homosexuality" (these positions identify homosexual practice as sin and bar "self-affirming, practicing" homosexuals from church office-- i.e., ordination). At the same time the letter noted that the issues raised by the majority report will not go away, including "the sexual *needs* of singles, gay and lesbian persons, the disabled, and older adults." The letter concluded with the reassertion, from the denomination's "historic principles" of 1788, that "God alone is Lord of the conscience" and that "there are truths and forms with respect to which people of deep faith may differ." My deep appreciation is extended to Dr. Kenneth Cuthbertson, Chicago, for the clarifying information for this note.

[4]For example studies, see: J. Michael Clark, *A defiant celebration: Theological ethics and gay sexuality* (Garland, TX: Tangelwüld Press, 1990) and *Masculine socialization and gay liberation: A conversation on the work of James Nelson and other wise friends* (with Bob McNeir; Dallas: Publishers Associates, under review [1992]).

[5]Clark, *A place, op cit.,* p. 1.

[6]Richard L. Rubenstein, *After Auschwitz: Radical theology and contemporary Judaism* (Indianapolis: Bobbs-Merrill, 1966), p. 246.

[7]Chaim Potok's novels, in order of first publication, include: *The chosen* (New York: A.A. Knopf, 1967), *The promise* (New York: A.A. Knopf, 1969), *My name is Asher Lev* (New York: A.A. Knopf, 1972. Fawcett-Crest edition, 1974), *In the beginning* (New York: A.A. Knopf, 1975), *The book of lights* (New York: A.A. Knopf, 1981), *Davita's harp* (New York: A.A. Knopf, 1985), and *The gift of Asher Lev* (New York: A.A. Knopf, 1990); his non-fiction historical volume is entitled: *Wanderings: Chaim Potok's history of the Jews* (New York: A.A. Knopf, 1978. Fawcett-Crest edition, 1984).

[8]Clark, *Masculine socialization, op cit.*

[9]Potok, *Wanderings, op cit.,* especially pp. 11-14.

[10]*Ibid.,* pp. 12-13.

[11]Clark, *Masculine socialization, op cit.*

[12]Cf., Clark, *A place, op cit.,* p. 61.

[13]Cf., *ibid.,* p. 67.

[14]Cf., *ibid.,* pp. 64-65.

[15]Cf., *ibid.,* p. 77.

[16]Cf., *ibid.*, p. 78.

[17]Cf., *ibid.*, p. 82.

[18]Cf., *ibid.*, p. 91.

[19]See: J. Michael Clark, *Defiant, op cit.*; *A lavender cosmic pilgrim: Further ruminations on gay spirituality, theology, and sexuality* (Las Colinas, TX: The Liberal Press, 1990), pp. 55-78; *Theologizing gay: Fragments of liberation activity* (Oak Cliff, TX: Minuteman Press, 1991), pp. 48-57; and, *Masculine socialization, op cit.*

[20]Cf., Clark, *Defiant, op cit.*, pp. 50-54; *Theologizing gay, op cit.*, p. 56f; and, *Masculine socialization, op cit.*

[21]Cf., Clark, *Lavender, op cit.*, pp. 7-39.

[22]Cf., John E. Fortunato, *AIDS, the spiritual dilemma* (San Francisco: Harper & Row, 1987).

[23]Raymond A. Moody, *Life after life* (New York: Bantam, 1975).

[24]The most notorious of more recent messianic pretenders within Judaism was Shabbetai Zevi (1626-1676); see: Potok, *Wanderings, op cit.*, pp. 446-454.

[25]For a poignant example of Christian antisemitism portrayed in fiction, see: Bernard Malamud, *The fixer* (New York: Farrar, Straus & Giroux, 1966).

[26]Cf., Clark, *A place, op cit.*, p. 116.

[27]Cf., *ibid.*, p. 104.

[28]Cf., *ibid.*, p. 105.

[29]Cf., *ibid.*, pp. 175-179.

[30]Cf., *ibid.*, pp. 104-107.

[31]Cf., *ibid.*, p. 178.

[32]This prayer was developed by the author in 1986 and subsequently used in the Shabbat evening service of Yom HaShoah remembrance at Atlanta's Congregation Bet Haverim, 1 May 1987. It draws upon both the traditional Reform movement prayerbook and the work of Richard Plant and others on the experience of gay men during the Holocaust. For examples, see: Richard Plant, *The pink triangle: The Nazi war against homosexuals* (New York: Henry Holt, 1986) and J. Michael Clark, *Pink triangles and gay images: (Re)claiming communal and personal history in retrospective gay fiction* (Arlington, TX:

Liberal Arts Press, 1987), pp. 15-35; this prayer was originally published as an Appendix in the latter volume, pp. 65-67.

[33]Between its founding in May 1985 and January 1987, the ritual committee of Congregation Bet Haverim (Atlanta) gradually pulled together the materials for what would then become the group's own congregationally-appropriate prayerbook. Synagogue members contributed materials from a wide range of places and resources, the original sources for which were most often no longer traceable. A number of prayers, however, did come from the prayerbooks of other gay/lesbian synagogues. In the January 1987 self-publication of that prayerbook, and here in this context as well, these established congregations are gratefully acknowledged for facilitating the early development of Congregation Bet Haverim and for contributing various ideas, translations, and readings for its prayerbook during its early years prior to affiliation with the Reconstructionist movement (1990): Congregation Beth Simchat Torah, New York; Congregation Sha'ar Zahav, San Francisco; and the Metropolitan Community Synagogue, Miami. My deep appreciation is extended to all four synagogues as the collective resource for those prayers which I have reconstructed herein; parenthetical citations are to the January 1987 version of the Congregation Bet Haverim prayerbook.

[34]The rationale and methodology for the paraphrases which follow are an extension of a method described by Marcia Falk, "Notes on composing new blessings," in *Weaving the visions: New patterns in feminist spirituality* (ed. J. Plaskow & C.P. Christ; San Francisco: Harper & Row, 1989), pp. 128-138.

[35]Morton, *op cit.* (n. 2, above).

[36]Sheila D. Collins, "Theology in the politics of Appalachian women," in *Womanspirit rising: A feminist reader in religion* (ed. C.P. Christ & J. Plaskow; San Francisco: Harper & Row, 1979), p. 152.

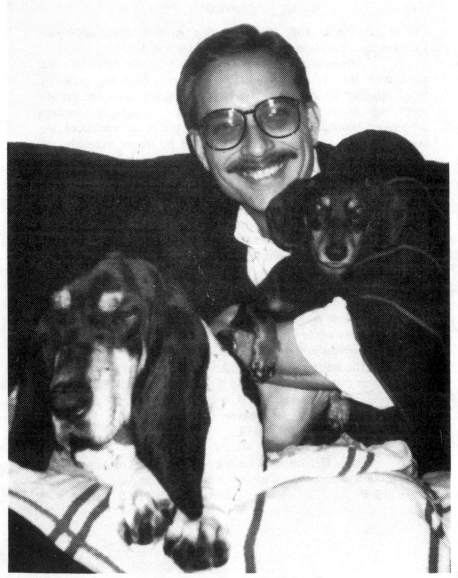

J. Michael Clark & Friends

V. Notes on Contributors

Ronald E. Long (Ph.D., Columbia University, 1985) now refers to himself as a New Yorker, since he has lived in New York City since he first started graduate study there in 1969. He was educated at Kenyon College in Ohio and at Columbia, and was for a year a Fulbright Scholar to then West Germany. He has taught at Vassar and at Columbia, and is now Adjunct Assistant Professor of Religion (part-time) at Hunter College/City University of New York--where he teaches, among others, courses on death, the religious dimensions of the erotic, and contemporary western thought. This book marks not only his publishing debut, but also his "coming out" in print. It is in part an answer to questions posed by the illness and death from AIDS of his first lover. He is now welcoming a new lover, Robert Pesce, into his life. Ron shares the fate of other unapologetic gay theologians in not having a full-time academic position, and supplements his income by working as a one-on-one personal trainer in a Manhattan gym.

J. Michael Clark (Ph.D., Emory University, 1983) is currently a free-lance scholar/writer/theologian who teaches freshmen English at Georgia State University and pre-freshmen writing and critical thinking at Emory University. He has published numerous books and articles in gay theology, ethics, and socioliterary criticism and is the founding co-convenor of the Gay Men's Issues in Religion Group of the American Academy of Religion. A native southerner who settled in Atlanta over a decade ago, he now lives with his spouse, Bob McNeir, and their dogs, "big sister" basset hound Abigail and "little sister" dachshund Little Bit.